USUI'S TEACHER

The Writings of Tanaka

The SECRETS of
Taireido and Reishi

With teachings on
spirituality, psychic, healing, and therapies

Forewords & footnotes
Frank Shortt
and
Allan Sweeney

USUI'S TEACHER - The Writings of Tanaka

By Frank Shortt & Allan Sweeney

'Heaven-by-the-Sea,' 5 Beach Houses,
Royal Crescent, Margate, Kent CT9 5AL United Kingdom

(Allan Sweeney's profits from this book help cancer research)

Published in the UK by Mastership Pathway UK
Printed in China by Chinee Printing Inc.
through Rei On International

978-0-9543726-4-4

DEDICATION

This book is dedicated to

Usui's Reiki

Tanaka's Taireido and Reishi

Usui's and Tanaka's quests for the purest spirituality

And Usui's and Tanaka's hope that scientific research can validate

Healing cures with their systems.

SPECIAL THANKS

I would like to take this opportunity to thank a few people that have been great guiding lights on my journey in life and in my search for knowledge. First and foremost, I thank my parents (you know who you are) who have been my biggest support and provided me with living examples of how one should live life in truth and love. My wife and her family, amazing as they all are. Dr. Allan Sweeney, for teaching and guiding me in my spiritual practice of Reiki, he has also been a true inspiration and driving force for this work to be completed. James Deacon, who has provided guidance in my further study of Reiki, its roots and its meanings from a sober and lucid point of view, and for his expertise in Japanese spirituality and cultural history.

Kind regards to you the reader, and all who have supported us in this process.

Frank Shortt

"A-Z" OF THANKS

Always thank Reiki for healing ourselves, friends, families, and patients

Blessedly thank spirituality enhanced by Reiki

Creatively thank how Reiki improves negative events, both near and far

Discoveries of new and better ways to use Reiki are thankfully received

Energetically, Reiki is thanked for inner and outer bio-field healings

Family love and thanks to parents Ted and Betty, and my daughter Angela.

Globe-trotting thanks that Reiki has travelled to heal poorer nations

Heart-felt thanks to my patients, students and friends around the world

(Do contact me if you need help again)

Injuries and injustices give thanks for Reiki

Jobs offering Reiki are gratefully thanked

Kindly thank Reiki for the gentle characteristics it produces within us

LOvingly thank Reiki that helps many without love find LOve

Measurements of outcomes are thanked, showing evidence that Reiki works

Nothing being beyond Reiki ability is thanked

Omnipotent powers of Godly Reiki potential are thanked

Pathways are thanked, as Reiki helps find our soul journeys on Earth

Quests are thanked, as Reiki unveils our spiritual and mystical paths

Research thanks that proves Reiki heals physical, emotions, mental spiritual

Souls are thanked, that are helped by Reiki especially when lost and alone

Therapies thank Reiki that can sometimes relieve suffering after doctors fail

Ultimate thanks for the greatest inclusion of Reiki with orthodox medicine

Validations that Reiki alleviates health conditions are academically thanked

Warm feelings of thanks to Reiki for its limitless ways to improve humanity

X-rays are thanked that show fractures, broken bones are healed by Reiki

Yahoo, Google, Internet Explorer are thanked for sending Reiki good news

Zeal and zest for life that Reiki provides are immensely thanked

And may I please thank Morihei Tanaka for his many writings, and dedication to the healing and spiritual movement; Dr Usui for starting the Reiki healing and spiritual system; Dr Hayashi for sharing Reiki in his clinic; Mrs Takata for teaching Reiki that spread globally; the guides and masters and angels and Gods who may be around, albeit unseen, to help millions of Reiki persons on their journey; the intelligent nature of the Reiki energy for the beauteous gifts it bestows on all; and the highest thanks of LOve that the bountiful wonder of Reiki energy will only ever be used for the highest good of all concerned.

Blessings of Reiki LOve

Allan Sweeney

Please visit
http://usuisteacher.com
Or my sites
www.reiki-healing.com
www.grecianreiki.com

CONTENTS

LIST OF ILLUSTRATIONS

PREFACE

By Frank Shortt

The discovery of Tanaka's Taireido and Reishi

The discovery of TAIREIDO and the work of Morihei Tanaka came to me by unexpected coincidence. It brought significant revelation to my understanding of the 'Reiki history', and insight into the foundation of the Reiki system.

The journey of discovery started with a Reiki-researcher, James Deacon, who knew of an Italian Reiki Practitioner and Martial Artist who had in his possession a Japanese copy of 'TAIREIDO; A New Revelation, The Spiritual, Mental and Physical Salvation of Mankind.' I subsequently tried to track down my own volume, and found only 3 other copies, one in New York, one in London, and one in Sidney – all home cities of prominent Theosophists. It may be seen from our footnotes in this book that perhaps some of Tanaka's roots might have connected to Theosophy teachings?

Luckily the 'Taireido' volumes were in English. Although no translation was needed, some spellings needed correction. The whole 447-page volume was transcribed by the end of December 2009 and is reprinted in this book in 10-point Times New Roman, to reduce the number of pages and keep the cost down for readers.

On the suggestion and encouragement from my wife, Joana Taya Borges da Silva; my brother in law, Tiago Borges da Silva; and my Reiki Master, Allan Sweeney; I decided to get the work published, together with Allan Sweeney, to benefit potentially all of Mankind, moreover ensuring the knowledge contained within these pages are carried forward to our future generations.

With the help of Allan's lovely Japanese friend Taeko Ono (married as Taeko Fleet), we discovered and bought two other volumes, written in Japanese, of work on Taireido written by Mr. Tanaka in 1916 and republished in 2001. Taeko confirmed those two volumes are almost the same as the book we are presenting here – it seems that substantially, this 1920 volume combines both 1916 Japanese volumes.

Through her research, Taeko became convinced that the book presented here is an English translation of Morihei Tanaka's publications concerning the doctrine of Taireido. It seems our English volume is unique, and published after the Japanese volumes, with slight adjustments to material.

Taeko found other volumes too, with the earliest writing dating back to 1910. She suggested that:

> "The 1920 [our edition] edition seem to be specially produced for Western readers, and I've got an impression that 1920 edition might be the translation of 'TAIREIDO SHINTEN' 1910 edition."[1]

On the investigation into the organisation Taireido Hojin established by Tanaka and who also published his work, she concluded the following:

> "TAIREIDO HONIN should correctly be TAIREIDO HOJIN (possible translation mistake), and HOJIN means a corporation.
>
> It's highly unlikely that the corporation is still active. In 1920, Tanaka built DAIHON-IN (the head quarters of his healing centre) but, it completely burnt down, and then in 1928 he died of heart disease. After his death, Taireido apparently died out and has been completely forgotten."[2]

On the possible influence of any earlier spiritual founder on Morihei Tanaka, she concluded with:

> "I haven't found another earlier spiritual founder, although there are a few contemporary founders."[3]

To supplement this information:

> **1911** - Tanaka established the Reiri Gakkai Tokyo (Tokyo Spiritualist Society).
>
> **1916** - Tanaka established HON-IN TAIREIDO, (the main temple of Taireido) in the Kojimachi area of Tokyo.
>
> **1920** Tanaka established ENA DAIHON-IN (The Great Monastery of Ena) in the village of Takenami.

Of the contemporary spiritual movements in the late 1800s and early 1900s, most notable is the Oomoto (foundation) movement. Also known as Ōmoto-kyō, it was founded by Deguchi Nao (1836-1918), and is categorized as a Japanese "New Religion" originating from Shinto.

[1-3] Taeko Fleet

From what I can gather it was the main competitor to the Taireido movement (also officially classified as a Shinto sect, or offshoot[4]).

The Oomoto movement and its spiritual teacher (seishi) Deguchi Onisaburō (1871-1948) was also responsible for encouraging Morihei Ueshiba (1883-1969), to develop Aikido. They also influenced the spiritual doctrine of the founder, who is often referred to as Kaiso or Chossô, meaning "founder", or Ōsensei, meaning "Great Teacher."

Mikao Usui, 15 August 1865 – 9 March 1926, was the founder of what we today know as Reiki Ryoho, or simply Reiki.

There are many similarities between all these founders and the practices they put forth. Especially noticeable is the spiritual enlightenment that was a precursor to the spiritual movement that followed from these founders.

At times these healing and spiritual practices are not just similar, but downright identical. Most notable is the similarity or identical nature between Reiki and Taireido, and that is what this book will attempt to point out.

This in no way discredits the practice of Reiki, but will in my opinion rather give the reader a better understanding of the practice. From commentary given in this book, it seems highly likely that the founder of Reiki, Mikao Usui, knew the practice of Reishi as referred to in the doctrine of Taireido, as there seems to be many similarities within these two systems.

Currently the 'proof' that Usui was a practitioner of Reishi and possibly even a follower of Taireido, is that both the teachings and the practice of Reiki can be found within the doctrine of Taireido and the practice of Reishi. As mentioned, at times the details of the practice of Taireido are identical to what we find in the practice of Reiki. Yet Taireido was written and published before Usui is known to have practiced Reiki.

It is also worth noting that the two founders, Tanaka and Usui came from the same area - Gifu prefecture, which is located just over half-ways from Tokyo to Kyoto. Mikao Usui's village is located just north of the city of Gifu and Morihei Tanaka´s village just east of the city, approximately 44 km from each other.

---

[4] "The Oxford handbook of global religions" -p.146, Mark Juergensmeyer, Oxford University Press; http://en.wikipedia.org/wiki/Shinto_sects_and_schools

By the time Usui-sensei had his enlightenment, satori or "kantoku," and developed what we know as Reiki, the practice of Reishi and the doctrine of Taireido was already very well known and practiced all over the country. Morihei Tanaka was also a high profile figure throughout Japan at the time, and it is without doubt that Usui would have known of him, his movement and the practice of Reishi.

Both founders also coined the term for their version of mysterious spiritual power almost the same;

Reishi = Spirit-force, Spiritual Strength or Spiritual Action;
Reiki = Spirit-force or Spiritual Action.

This will be further discussed in the chapters concerning Reishi.

It is also possible that Usui became familiar with and studied the practice of Reishi from the many publications that the organisation put out to the public, and did not attend the Reishi "seminars." This we leave to the readers' rationale.

This volume, 'Taireido: A New Revelation for the Spiritual, Mental and Physical Salvation of Mankind', by Tanaka Morihei, founder of Taireido, was published in 1920 by Taireido Hojin. According to Tanaka himself, it is the complete thought and practice of the system, and seems to be a compilation of earlier publications by Tanaka.

So far we have found, thanks to Taeko Fleet, 11 other publications by Tanaka, (2 of the books published in 1916, republished 2001):

(1) "TAIREIDO SHINTEN" (1910) [Reprinted edition in 1954]

(2) "TENSHIN SIJO TAIREI SHINTEN" (1911)

(3) "TAIREIDO OYOBI REISIJUTSU KOJUROKU Vol. 1-2" (1916) [Reprinted edition 2001]

(4) "TAIREIDO NO HONGI" (1918)

(5) "TAIREIDO SHUGENDEN" (1918)

(6) "TAIREIDO - A new revelation showing the true system of life; an outline only" (1919)

(7) "TAIREIDO - A new revelation for the spiritual, mental and physical salvation of mankind" (1920) The book presented herein

(8) "TAIREIDO GAKUBUMON Vol.1 - 2" (1921-22)

(9) "TAIREIDO REISHIJUTSU KOUJUROKU Vol.1 - 2"
apparently reprinted edition of (7), published by Sengabo

(10) "TAIREIDO REISHIJUTSU KOUJUROKU Vol.1 - 2"
published by Hachiman Shoten

Commentaries on Taireido:

(11) "TAIREIDO - Methods of developing super power" by Ikko Takagi

Even if Taireido and the practice of Reishi is not the precursor to Reiki, it still gives a great insight into the Reijutsu (spiritual art, spiritual skill) movement of the time of Mikao Usui, which Reiki was most definitely a later part of.

Nowadays in the 21st century, we see many 'different' healing modalities, which at their core are very similar or even identical. It is more often than not the founder's personality that sets systems apart. Also nowadays it can be seen that different modalities "borrow" from each others' theory, philosophy and practices. I do not think it was much different in Usui or Tanaka's time.

At any rate, over the years, Morihei Tanaka and Taireido have been mentioned as the precursor to Reiki, and even that Tanaka was Usui's teacher. We have not found any concrete proof of this, and therefore will not make such a claim; but there are many things that make it highly likely that Tanaka was, directly or indirectly, Usui's teacher. However, we will rather let the reader make his or her own mind up regarding whether Tanaka had direct or indirect or no influence on Usui's teachings and will proceed to deliver what we found in the work of Morihei Tanaka and how it relates to Reiki.

Brief bio history of Morihei Tanaka (1884 - 1928)

He was born 8, September 1884, in the Ena district, Gifu-prefect. He was either born in the village of Tajimi or Takenami close to Usui-sensei's birthplace, Miyama-Cho.

He was a primary school teacher, and worked in the Press Office of the Ministry of Finance in Tokyo. It was during this time that his life would change drastically.

The setting: "The Sino-Japanese War of 1894, was ended, but with the Japanese armies of occupation still in Korea and southern Manchuria. Russia demanded the retrocession of the Liaotung Peninsula from Japan. In

1897, a Russian squadron anchored at Port Arthur. In the immediate years leading up to 1902, the Japanese had made an alliance with Britain and Russian. The Japanese diplomats made a series of agreements about Korea and Manchuria, but Russia broke the agreements, and occupied Manchuria.

Morihei Tanaka was very passionate and patriotic, and to him, the Russian occupation of Manchuria was a major threat to the sovereignty of the Empire of Japan. In his passion for the Empire, he wrote an appeal to the Emperor to go to war against this threat. He then handed his appeal to the Emperor himself, which got him arrested and sent back to his village under house-arrest. Soon after, on the 8, February 1904, Japan issued a declaration of war. Some observers of the day thought Tanaka had influenced the decision for war, and he became nationally famous.

During his time of "arrest" he dedicated himself to study and spiritual discipline, and moved into the mountains of Gifu. It was during this time of spiritual discipline and fasting, that he received enlightenment (Satori or Kantoku) and understood the truth of Tairei (the Great Spirit). This came about after four months of spiritual discipline which involved fasting and isolation in the mountain, and through this discipline he developed *Reishiryoku* (special powers).

He then went on to study and develop the doctrine of Taireido (The Way of the Great Spirit) and *Reishijutsu* - the art of Reishi. By the end of the Russo-Japanese war he had become well known for his spiritual powers and his healing abilities and established the Taireido Hojin.

The Legacy of Morihei Tanaka had begun, and soon spread throughout Japan, and into China and Mongolia. It is even speculated and claimed by some that Morihei Tanaka had a great influence on Chinese Qi-Gong.

FOREWORD

By Frank Shortt

Taireido: Relationship to Reiki

This foreword is a detailed introduction to the system of healing, spirituality and thought called TAIREIDO, and the practice of the art of REISHI and the effects of REISHI ACTION. The aims are:

1. To suggest some of the writings and thoughts that may link teachings and ideas of Dr Mikao Usui with Morihei Tanaka; and

2. To suggest further links in a lineage from Morihei Tanaka, Mikao Usui, Chijiro Hayashi and Hawayo Takata, to modern masters.

In Japan in March 1922[5], on a spiritual mountain near Kyoto called Kurama Yama, Dr Mikao Usui is said to have undergone strict spiritual discipline and meditated, perhaps for 21 days. This is said to have resulted in him achieving enlightenment as a visionary mystical experience. This enlightenment has been called '*satori*', a common term in Japanese spiritual practice, or '*kantoku*' a term used in some Shinto schools of practice.

According to convention, during this experience on the mountain Usui acquired what he called 'a spiritual gift', which referred to his newfound abilities to heal. According to Mrs Takata, when he came down the mountain, he cured a young girl's toothache, and started offering lectures. Consequently, it is told that Usui thus developed his spiritual system, his reiho, and became a sensei. Today, Usui-sensei's system is called 'Usui Reiki Ryoho' or simply 'Reiki.'

(Strangely, as is shown later in this book, Morihei Tanaka is described as having an almost identical experience, including receiving enlightenment on a mountain, and being shown how to heal, and healing toothache after, and then giving lectures on the subject – yet this was a number of years before Usui discovered Reiki.)
In the mid-late 1990s some documents surfaced from Japan, presumably being Usui-sensei's own words describing his Reiki Therapy, a Q&A, and a

---

[5] Some claim that Usui-sensei had his mystical experience or enlightenment in 1914, although it is commonly thought that it was not until 1922 that Usui-sensei achieved this. However, one of Tanaka's books was published around 1910, predating Usui by between four to twelve years.

treatment guide ('*Shishin*'). Allan Sweeney was the first person from outside Japan to be invited to Japan to address the inaugural meeting of Japanese Reiki masters and senseis in Tokyo and receive Dr Usui's writings. These documents, under the name '*Hikkei*', were apparently compiled by Hoichi Wanami-sensei, the 5th President of Usui Reiki Gakkai, which was Usui's Reiki Organisation/Society. This Gakkai was created by Usui-sensei and was continued by his students after his death, until today. Very little is known of this society and hence conspiracy theories around this 'secret society' have been rampant since the late '90s.

As the 'Hikkei' is written in the first person and gives Usui-sensei as the writer, it is commonly assumed it was either written by him directly or by someone he met, perhaps a reporter or student who recorded his words. So one way or another the '*Hikkei*' is probably a direct record of Usui-sensei's words. One of Usui-sensei's students, Hayashi-sensei, compiled his own treatment guide (Hayashi Reiki Shishin as opposed to Usui Reiki Shishin), which is very similar to Usui-sensei's guide.

In 'The Explanation of Usui Therapy' found at the start of the '*Hikkei*', Usui-sensei discusses the origin of the system we know as Reiki.

> "The Usui Reiki Therapy is something no one before has discovered, and bears comparison with no other treatment in the world. On this understanding, we make known the Reiki Therapy for the benefit of the public in the hope that many people will receive Heaven's blessing, ensuring the unity of body and soul, thereby enjoying natural welfare. From its origins, the Usui Reiki Therapy has been an innovative spiritual therapy based on universal spiritual powers."
>
> *Reiki Hikkei - Explanation of Usui Therapy*[6]

This statement sounds very much like the proclamations made by Morihei Tanaka, founder of Taireido, a system of thought predating Usui-sensei's Reiho (Reiki Ryoho). As we shall see through this book, these two systems are very similar, and even use similar statements, proclamations, phrases, and sentences. Similar to Usui-sensei, Tanaka also fasted and had undergone strict spiritual discipline in the mountains, in 1904/1905, and published his first work in 1910, and started Reiri Gakkai Tokyo (Tokyo Spiritualist Society) 1911.

---

[6] Dr. Allan Sweeney "Explanation of Reiki Therapy" © 1998, and "The Reiki 1 Manual" © 2002

Having said that, there are of course points that differ in the two systems, but perhaps only similar to the differences of students in modern lineages to the teachings of their masters! But the similarities are so profound and often so repetitious, that there is good reason to believe that Usui-sensei's system is heavily influenced by, or a continuation of, the work of Tanaka.

The first part of Tanaka's book is an in-depth introduction to his system of thought, coined as Taireido and the Art of Reishi Action.

Tanaka starts his work by proclaiming TAIREIDO as transcending all religions, ethics and morality. This seems an attempt to place his system of thought, Taireido, as the forerunner, essence or foundation of non-religious spiritual systems. He gives a rather lengthy discourse explaining his stance on these subjects and the superiority of his newfound system of thought, which he considers the salvation of Mankind.

> 'Taireido comprehends yet transcends philosophy, ethics and religion.'
>
> Morihei Tanaka, TAIREIDO

Reiki embraces similar teachings regarding religion. Reiki is not a religion, and it can work with all faiths. One does not need to believe, one may understand spirituality by experiencing the effects. The effects include healing of others, as shown in this questions and answer.

> Q: Cannot illness be cured without believing in the Usui Reiki Therapy?
>
> A: Unlike psychological treatment, hypnotherapy and other mental treatments, the Usui Reiki Therapy does not bring with it empty implications[7]. It does not therefore require an explicit consent on the part of the patient[8] or any loyalty to the practitioner concerned. Not only that, we practitioners of the Usui Reiki Therapy do not mind however much our practices are doubted, held in contempt or rejected[9]. For example, the Usui Reiki Therapy is remarkably effective in treating even those who are unconscious of the world around them,

---

[7] Highly knowledgeable, Dr Usui was not averse to being blunt and tough to impart his message.

[8] Contrary to many books Dr Usui says categorically that patients do not have to give permission

[9] Patients do not have to believe in Reiki.

> such as infants and patients with serious diseases[10]. People, who believe in, admire and respect our therapy with only the first treatment, would number one in ten, if that[11]. Many such people appreciate for the first time, upon being treated once, the efficacy of the Usui Reiki Therapy, and all at once, they begin to trust it.
>
> Reiki Hikkei[12]

Tanaka makes the same claims through this book. The two main documents that give us an insight into Usui-sensei's history, his spiritual system (Reiki) and its practice are: 'The Reiki Hikkei', and the Memorial Stone found at Usui-sensei's grave. There are also Japanese teachings that have come through lineages such as those starting with Hayashi - Takata, Hayashi - Yamaguchi, or Kondo - Doi.

The teachings of Reiki seem identical to Taireido in transcending religion. As for morality and ethics, Reiki seems to have very similar effects to that alluded to by Tanaka. Both Tanaka and Usui's students pointed out that the world has continued its downward spiral and how Reiki or Taireido could change this.

This shows the similarities in the philosophy of the two systems, namely Usui Reiho and Morihei Tanaka's Taireido.

A reference to the world situation that seems to agree with Tanaka's sentiment is written by one of Japans well known memorial text composers, Masayuki Okada, on Usui-sensei's Memorial Stone.

> "Recently the state of the world has altered and peoples' thoughts have changed a great deal. Hopefully, the spread of this Spiritual Method will be of great help to people who have a confused mind or who do not have morality. Surely it is not only of benefit in curing chronic diseases and lingering complaints?"
>
> Masayuki Okada, Doctor of Literature,
> Subordinate 3rd rank, 3rd Order of Merit.[13]

---

[10] Patients do not even have to know that Reiki is being given - for Reiki still works effectively.

[11] Showing possibly a similar reaction to present-day patients.

[12] Dr. Allan Sweeney "Explanation of Reiki Therapy" © 1998, and "The Reiki 1 Manual" © 2002

[13] James Deacon's Translation by Jiro Kozuki for http://aetw.org

Reishi, Taireido and Divinity are topics that crop up several times in Tanaka's book. Tanaka emphasizes time and again that his method allows one's own divinity to touch the divinity of another, and when this occurs healing takes place as described in this book.

> 'We believe that the universe is the product of one principle called *Reishi* which is an emanation of *Tairei* true and good.'
>
> Morihei Tanaka, TAIREIDO

'The Divine Spark' or one's own divinity, is a topic that seems to come up for discussion quite often amongst contemporary Reiki Practitioners and Masters in public forums, like the Reiki Learning Lounge. The notion that Reiki (like Tanaka's notion of Taireido, or Reishi) is the divinity within us and all of creation seems to come close to how modern practitioners feel about the Reiki phenomena. This seems to be reflected in Tanaka's words here:

> "By TAIREIDO a man becomes able to express the divinity within him, letting it shine forth in glowing radiance upon the world. A careful perusal of the following pages will indicate in some measure how this is true."
>
> Morihei Tanaka, TAIREIDO

As shown by Tanaka's various publications and translations to English, his mission was to spread this gift to benefit society, the nation, and all Mankind. This is clearly stated at the start of this volume, and emphasized throughout.

> "Once TAIREIDO is studied and apprehended the meaning of Man's life at last becomes plain, **his thought is unified and he has permanent peace of mind**."
>
> Morihei Tanaka, TAIREIDO

Tanaka is clearly very passionate in that his system of thought would benefit society and the nation, as well as all of Mankind. He shows himself to be a man of the nation, deeply concerned with the well-being of his fellow men. There are similar points in the writings of Usui-sensei as found in the '*Hikkei.*'

> "...we make known the Reiki Therapy for the benefit of the public in the hope that many people will receive Heaven's blessing, ensuring the unity of body and soul, thereby enjoying natural welfare. From its origins, the Usui Reiki Therapy has been an innovative spiritual therapy based on universal spiritual powers. First of all, therefore, it

makes persons healthy, and at the same time improves their mind, thereby improving mankind's enjoyment of human life.

This is why I take it upon myself to proclaim the Usui Reiki Therapy to my fellow creatures who require some relief from illnesses that are giving them pain both internally and externally."

Usui-sensei, 'Reiki Hikkei:
Explanation of Reiki Therapy'[14]

From this translation of the '*Hikkei*', one can see that the sentiments of the Founders of Taireido and Reiki are almost identical. The more one studies the texts, and practices the methods described, the more one is led to believe that Usui-sensei echoes Morihei Tanaka on most accounts.

It is known to us through the teachings of Reiki Ryoho, and the Memorial Stone found at Usui-sensei's grave that he was committed to rigorous discipline and studied hard. Because Tanaka's works were famous in Japan, and were published a few years before Usui's enlightenment, it is highly unlikely that Tanaka's Taireido and the Art of Reishi Action had not been studied by Usui, at least to some degree.

Especially it should be noted that the Taireido movement enjoyed wide popularity throughout Japan. This book shows that the similarities in teaching, philosophy, and practice of the two systems, are profound. So it seems likely that Taireido predates Reiki by just a few years, and was still being taught when Usui started teaching. It is therefore most likely that Usui-sensei understood Tanaka's approaches.

In regard to the practice of Reiki, it requires certain careful preparation of mind and body, similar to the preparation necessary and outlined by Tanaka in the chapters that follow. One can often hear Reiki practitioners referring to this with language such as 'getting out of the way, so that Reiki may flow', or 'connect to Reiki' (sometimes called the 'highest source'). Usually Reiki is taught and seen/felt as coming from high above, flowing into and through the practitioner to the recipient. Even more, one is usually taught different preparatory techniques to relax the body and the mind before engaging in the practice of Reiki. These all seem to connect current Reiki practices with methods of Tanaka in this book.

[14] Dr. Allan Sweeney "Explanation of Reiki Therapy" © 1998, and "The Reiki 1 Manual" © 2002

Similarly Usui yet again echoes Tanaka on the need to have medical knowledge in order to do 'Usui's reiho' effectively, and in applying Reiki direct to certain body parts.

> "Since our therapy is a spiritualistic method of therapy that has transcended modern science, it is not based on medicine. Simply, if the patient suffers pain in the chest, the practitioner of this therapy considers the patient's chest, if the stomach gives pain, then the stomach, and if there is something wrong with the eyes, then the practitioner must be concerned with the patient's eyes themselves. In this way, the therapy achieves its objective of curing solely through a steady gaze on the diseased area, breathing on it, the laying-on of hands or stroking. Therefore, there is no need for the patient to take bitter medicine or be subjected to blisteringly hot moxa cautery, and in a short time the said diseases will be cured. This is the reason for this unique spiritualistic therapy [reiho]."
>
> Usui-sensei, Usui Reiki Hikkei Q&A[15]

Many Reiki practitioners accept that if the body is tense or stressed, it will hinder the 'flow' or action of Reiki. The same goes for the mind that is not at ease. Hence the preparatory techniques taught to me by Sweeney were in three steps.

1. Calm the breath
2. Calm the body
3. Calm the mind

These points are also emphasized in Taireido, as part of the preparations necessary for Reishi Treatment, thus connecting certain modern Reiki practices to Tanaka. Tanaka also includes the eyes in his list, as he believes the eyes reflect the body and mind. This was also taught in my Reiki training with Sweeney.

Many Reiki masters suggest that, after a peaceful state has been achieved, one is ready to engage and 'connect' to the Reiki. To me these preparatory techniques seem very much in place to first set the right conditions in both body and mind for the practice to be effective. Second the techniques help put the practitioner in a state of transcendence, by connecting to something greater than oneself. I was also taught not to be attached to results while

---

[15] Dr. Allan Sweeney "Explanation of Reiki Therapy" © 1998, and "The Reiki 1 Manual" © 2002

doing the practice, as an 'attached mind' will hinder the efficiency of the practice. Taireido teaches in very similar ways. So with Taireido and Reiki, there is an emphasis on fluidity and effortless doing as opposed to stagnation and forceful tension, thus connecting the two systems.

These thoughts are also documented by the Taoist sages as the concept of 'wu-wei-wu', doing by not-doing, or 'by doing no-thing, everything is done.' Taoist thought has had a major influence on the spiritual (religious) and cultural aspects and development in Japan.

Tanaka lists a set of mental qualities one should foster in oneself to achieve greater proficiency in the Art of Reishi Action. In Usui Reiki Ryoho, there is no such list per se that has been discovered so far. However these qualities are emphasized directly or indirectly through teachings and practice. The following statement from Morihei Tanaka is very much in line with how I was taught Reiki, thus linking modern and ancient practices.

> "The timid and doubting practitioner will never attain results in applying the Art of Reishi."
>
> Morihei Tanaka, TAIREIDO

At the core of the Reiki teachings, we find a set of principals or precepts that seem to encompass Tanaka's list of mental virtues and Taireido's precepts. Usui-sensei himself put a lot of faith into the precepts as we can clearly see here in his words.

> "Shôfuku no hihô, Manbyo no rei yaku,
> Kyo dake wa
> Okoru na (ikaru na)
> Shinpai su na
> Kansha shite
> Gyo wo hage me
> Hito ni shinsetsu ni
> Asa you gassho shite kokoro ni nenji kuchi ni tonaeyo
> Shin shin kaizen
>
> Usui Reiki Ryoho
> Chossô, Usui Mikao"

Translated, we can read the importance Usui-sensei seems to have given these guidelines.

> "The Secret Method of inviting Happiness, The Miracle Medicine for all Illnesses.
> Just for today.

Do not have anger.
Do not worry.
Be full of gratitude.
Do your work honestly.
Be kind to all people,
Each morning and at night time, with hands held in prayer (gassho),
Think these in your mind and chant these with your mouth.
The Usui Reiki method brings cures to your mind and your body.

Usui Spiritual Healing Method
The founder, Mikao Usui"[16]

There are also a growing number of Reiki practitioners worldwide who are looking closer at the teachings of Takata-sensei.

> "In order to concentrate, one must purify one's thoughts in words, and to meditate to let true "energy" come out from within. It lies in the bottom of the stomach about 2 inches below the navel."
>
> *Takata-sensei's Diaries, December 10, 1935*[17]

The '*hara*' (litt. belly), more specifically the 'Seika Tanden'[18] play a major role in the respective practices. It seems like both Taireido and Reiki are no exception to this. Seika Tanden may also be known as '*Kikai Tanden*' - ocean of ki, and '*Seika no Itten*' - the One Point below the Navel.

> "By placing effortless emphasis and energy at this area in the lower abdomen, integration of body and mind is deepened and strengthened, and the Spirit is dynamically grounded in the Present Moment"[19]

The 'Seika Tanden' is considered by Tanaka and modern masters to be where one's life force is sd, even where one's spirit and soul reside. It is also the body's physical centre of gravity.

One can easily see the connection to the teachings of Tanaka, who also put great emphasis on this region of the body, and are reflected in his words here.

---

[16] Dr. Allan Sweeney "Gokai" © 1998, and "The Reiki 1 Manual" © 2002

[17] http://aetw.org/Reiki_takata_taught.htm

[18] Seika - below the navel; Tanden - field of the elixir.

[19] Japanese Reiki Techniques, http://aetw.org (Translations of Japanese terms also found there.)

> "Proper diaphragm tension is necessary to induction of full Reishi energy; in fact it is the source of such energy, and thereby one effects a proper application of the Reishi method. The abdomen is the seal of all spiritual power and action; and the more one has command of diaphragm action the more successful will one be in the application of the Art of Reishi."
>
> Morihei Tanaka, TAIREIDO

This is on par with Takata-sensei's emphasis of the '*hara*' or '*Seika Tanden*', and gives us a great clue to secrets of the art.

Concerning the treatment of disease, we shall again see that both Reiki and Reishi Action follow the same principals.

Reiki and Reishi are methods of healing as well as spiritual systems. Mr. Tanaka describes different methods of treating disease, similar to how I was taught to treat and practice Reiki. Tanaka, like Usui-sensei, Hayashi-sensei and my teacher Sweeney, presents a comprehensive treatment guide, listing many common diseases and specific treatment methods to achieve cures. Usui-sensei and Hayashi-sensei's treatment guides were said to be handed out to their students. We know them as 'Usui Ryoho Shishin' and 'Hayashi Ryoho Shishin.' These two documents are very similar, but nevertheless show a systematic approach to treatment, highlighting the most effective methods for treating specific diseases.

We know that Takata-sensei got Hayashi-sensei's 'Shishin' sometime from 1938 to 1940 from Hayashi-sensei himself, and has given it to at least some of her master students. In 1938 Takata received Master Level Certificate from Hayashi, and the last time they met was in 1940. On a side note, it also seems now that the common belief that Takata-sensei didn't teach for 35-years (1938-1973), Fran Brown being initiated to Reiki 1 in 1973, might now not hold up. At least one source[20], from Hawaii, has come forth and was apparently taught Reiki by Takata-sensei in the 1950s. It is more the case that she didn't start teaching master level students until the 70s.

She taught Reiki 1 & 2 to an unknown number of people, including her sister. Hayashi spoke of this in the radio interview he did when travelling and promoting Reiki in Hawaii. We are still waiting to hear if more information comes forth from this unnamed source, and I would keep an eye on the website referred to for updates on this. Through this source it might

---

[20] James Deacon, Research Pre-Fran Brown initiation. http://www.aetw.org/Reiki_takata_students.html

also be that the common idea that Reiki represents 'Universal Energy' might not have been introduced until the late 60's to fit the conceptual framework of the time. This doesn't mean much more than that it probably wasn't talked about in such a manner before the 1960s, hence other words might have been used to describe what the Reiki phenomena was.

This is an interesting point to note as we study the work of Morihei Tanaka. One can imagine that Usui-sensei might have used similar words to Tanaka to express his system and the phenomena that is Reiki. We shall see from the little writings and references to Usui-sensei that this does seem to be true – in fact in many cases, the words are almost identical.

These treatment guides (Usui/Hayashi & Tanaka) could only have come together by keeping patient records and noting the most effective treatment method for each particular disease. Like Tanaka, Usui-sensei notes that most disorders will be healed within a session of treatment, but chronic disease will most likely take multiple sessions. This again shows great concurrence between the two systems, Taireido & Reiki. Upon being asked if Usui's Reiki Ryoho was a spiritual healing method, Usui-sensei answers:

> "The Usui Reiki Therapy may certainly be termed a spiritualistic method of curing, but many of the aspects of the therapy may be called material therapy. The practitioner radiates a spirit and light from every part of his or her body. This spirit and light are manifested mostly in the eyes, the mouth and the hands. For this reason, the practitioner will carefully study the diseased part of the body for two or three minutes, breathe back on the patient, or massage the patient with the hands. By these means, inflammation will recede from the sites of tooth-ache, abdominal pain, gastro-enteritis, neurological pain, mastitis, scars, burns, and other sites of swelling. Chronic illnesses, however, may not be dealt with in this way, but I remember some cases of chronic illnesses which, usually requiring several sessions of treatment, have been successfully treated with just one session of Usui Reiki Therapy.
>
> How to explain this kind of phenomenon to modern medicinal circles? The facts of the account would sound more fantastic than the contents of a novel. However, if those actively interested in the teachings take a real look at the text, I believe they will assent to the assertions of those teachings. No matter how much the wordsmith may use sophistry in his art, he cannot deride the truth"

Usui-sensei, 'Reiki Ryoho Hikkei Q&A.' [21]

Individual, Group, and treatment at a distance, are set by Tanaka as the three ways of effecting a treatment using Reishi Action. This echoes in the modern Reiki practice as well. Most modern Reiki practitioners will be familiar with these methods as they have passed down from Usui-sensei - Hayashi-sensei - Takata-sensei in the form of "Teate (hands-on healing), Shuchu Reiki (Group Treatment), and Enkaku Chiryo ho (distance treatment).

While studying with Hayashi-sensei, Takata-sensei observed the regular employment of Group-Treatment in his clinic. Today Group Treatment is usually done in two ways, just as passed down from Hayashi-sensei. In one method a group of Reiki practitioners treat an individual, each one treating a different part of the body simultaneously.

Individual Treatment and Distance treatment will be familiar to most, if not all modern Reiki practitioners. All 2nd level (Okuden level) Reiki practitioners will be familiar with these practices.

Tanaka mentions the importance in keeping 'Patient Records,' a practice that Hayashi-sensei is known to have kept. I would also mention Allan Sweeney, as an example of 'modern' Reiki masters that practice similar methods of keeping records.

To me this is indicative of a system that is systematically upholding medical, scientific, and academic protocols (of the day) to improve the effectiveness of the treatment processes.

In this respect both founders, Morihei Tanaka and Mikao Usui, as well as some modern Reiki practitioners follow the same tradition. It may also show the possibility that the standards of Morihei Tanaka was passed on to Usui-sensei.

In treating disease by the Action of Reishi Tanaka lists four forms or techniques utilized to affect a cure. In Usui-sensei's explanation of Reiki Ryoho, he also mentions four techniques for *'teate'* treatment. Some of these methods are similar to ampuku or shiatsu massage techniques, which are traditional Japanese therapeutic practices. Shiatsu is well known now and was developed out of the Ampuku system.

---

[21] Dr. Allan Sweeney "Explanation of Reiki Therapy" © 1998, and "The Reiki 1 Manual" © 2002

"Ampuku (äm·pōō·kōō)
N.pr is a form of abdominal massage developed in Japan from Chinese sources, in which palpation of the abdomen (hara) is used for both the diagnosis and treatment of health complaints. This is also called Japanese abdominal massage."[22]

"Shiatsu
This is a Japanese form of acupressure involving finger pressure at specific points on the body, mainly for the purpose of balancing energy in the body."[23]

Here is a modern description of the Reiki techniques that are found within *'Teate.'*

"**Uchi te** involves tapping with the fingertips, or patting (not slapping) with the hands, using a light to medium force. The technique is an 'opening' one - applied to help stimulate and encourage energy flow and may be utilized at areas of blockage, inhibition or stagnation.

Oshi te involves pushing with the palms/'heel' of the hands or with the fingertips.

Oshi te is a 'loosening' technique - applied at areas of stiffness / tightness.

Nade te involves stroking or brushing in linear or circular direction with the hands. Like Uchi te, Nade te is an 'opening' technique - applied to help stimulate and encourage energy flow.

In using any of these techniques, one should be aware of Reiki flowing into the area being worked on." [24]

'Teate' is a hands-on healing treatment as known from modern Reiki healing.

In some countries today, there are laws that regulate 'touch' or 'manipulative' therapies such as Massage Therapy, therefore unless you are a licensed massage therapist, you may not legally use "Uchi te, Oshi te and Nade te" directly on the client in regions where these laws apply. But, the

[22] Mosby's Dictionary of Complementary and Alternative Medicine. © 2005, Elsevier.

[23] Mosby's Medical Dictionary, 8th edition. © 2009, Elsevier.

[24] James Deacon, Reiki Pages, © 2003, http://aetw.org/d_uon_te.html

techniques may be applied to the energy field instead of directly on the body.

Self-treatment is evident in both Usui-sensei's Reiki Ryoho and in Tanaka's Taireido. In the Art of Reishi as in Reiki, you would treat yourself as you would treat others; or you would treat others in the same manner as you treat yourself.

However, there is an apparent discrepancy in the teachings of Usui-sensei and Tanaka's Taireido, or so it would at least appear. Tanaka's teachings differentiate 'External Action of Reishi' and 'Internal Action of Reishi.' This distinction is not clearly found in Reiki. However, this distinction is common in both modern and ancient practice of healing. It can be seen in both Japanese energy modalities as well as Chinese/Taoist teachings on Qi, and in modern thoughts of energy coming down from an external source above and outside the head, (EXTERNAL) and energy moving inside a body to heal (INTERNAL). This coming together of External and Internal Reishi/Reiki is according to Tanaka what facilitates the healing effect. It may be seen as similar to the image of Heaven and Earth uniting in man.

The bodily reactions to the effects of 'External Reishi Action' as described by Tanaka are quite extreme, and there are cases of such severe reactions in relation to 'the Action of Reiki.' Some modern practitioners might suggest that Reiki works mostly akin to 'Internal Reishi Action' than to 'External Action of Reishi.' Involuntary movements of the body, such as a twitch of the leg or arm, shaking and similar have been found to occur in Reiki practitioners and their clients. Such reactions have also been mentioned by Tanaka in relation to Internal Reishi Action in patients receiving treatment, but that does not exclude External Action also being a cause that has similar potential effects. Tanaka states that, 'External Action of Reishi' is not effective in treating others, although some modern practitioners might suggest 'External Action' can have such effects...

In transmission of 'Internal Action of Reishi' Tanaka identifies that when a student has mastered both the 'Internal and External action of Reishi' it is always active in the practitioner and issues forth unconsciously without any intention to produce it. This is familiar to modern Reiki practices - when Reiki is acquired, it can flow continuously without effort from the practitioner and is sometimes referred to as 'intelligent' nature of Reiki. Similarly, Tanaka says at this level of skill, all one does is assume the proper state of mind and body and apply the finger or palm, and the internal action of Reishi will be transmitted. This sounds very familiar to Reiki.

It is in the practice and application of Reiki and Reishi one can see that the systems really start to merge.

Tanaka said that to fully grasp the action of Reishi, one should aim to have a similar experience of enlightenment as he had. By communing with nature, and undergoing spiritual discipline in forests and mountains. Maybe not coincidently, this is precisely what Usui-sensei did when he had his satori and experienced the phenomena of Reiki. The source of this information is written in stone, and can be found on Usui-sensei's Memorial Stone, where it states that Usui experienced '...a great Reiki over his head.'[25] This was a '*satori*' (enlightenment) or '*kantuko*' (Litt. realization or inspired vision) Therefore although Reiki and Taireido systems stand on their own, the more you study The Art of Reishi, the harder it is to think that Usui Reiki Ryoho was developed independently and ignorant of the teachings of Tanaka.

Usui, like Tanaka taught a basic formula of hand positions to be applied to the patient at the start of each treatment regardless of ailment. Each hand position is applied for two to three minutes in both systems, and after such application the treatment would proceed depending on need and severity of ailment. Both Usui and Tanaka had almost identical systems of therapy.

The method for generating 'Reishi Action' through mental focus, hand gestures, and deep diaphragmatic breathing was apparently practiced by ancient Japanese warriors, and is still practiced today in some schools of ninjutsu. However this breathing method potentially strains the physical body, so Tanaka suggests it should perhaps only be practiced with proper and gradual training.

As noted above Tanaka and Takata speak about the abdomen as the source of spiritual action or the source of Reishi/Reiki. Potentially, Takata learned this from her teacher Hayashi, back to Usui, and further back to Tanaka?

At any rate, many Reiki practitioners believe an energy centre exists deep inside your 'hara' (lower part of the abdomen), 3-4 cm below the navel. It is considered the focal point of all energies, personal, spiritual, physical, etc., etc. Traditional Japanese disciplines tend to speak of a single tanden.

> "However, in Japan there are also several disciplines - either of Chinese origin or alternatively heavily influenced by Chinese Chi Gung philosophy - which speak of three tandens:

[25] Usui's Memorial Stone translation

The Lower (Shimo) Tanden (also: Ge Tanden)
[essentially the same as the seika tanden]
- located deep inside the 'hara'

The Middle (Naka) Tanden (also: Chu Tanden)
- located inside the chest at about the heart level

The Upper (Kami) Tanden (also: Jo Tanden) - located in the middle of the head between the eyes"

James Deacon, Reiki Page © 2005

http://www.aetw.org/d_seika_tanden.html

In Reiki practice, just like the practice of 'the Art of Reishi Action,' there is no difference in treating others or oneself. There are also set hand-positions and treatment specifications that have come down to us from Usui-sensei - Hayashi-sensei - Takata-sensei and to contemporary Reiki Masters.

"Q: So, I can heal other people with it, but can I also heal myself?

A: If we can't heal our own disorders, how could we heal others?"

Reiki Hikkei Q&A

Takata-sensei and Tanaka are both known for believing that the best practice for Reiki or Reishi, and progress in the art, is by doing treatments.

Tanaka and Usui use almost identical language when stating that Reishi/ Reiki transcends modern science and provide a platform for curing mental and emotional problems/diseases.

Tanaka, being pragmatic, sees difficulty for a mentally ill person to treat himself or herself from a disease they might not even recognise. My teacher also taught this, but no Usui records claim either way. It would be interesting to know what Usui taught on this point, as Usui was pragmatic too, and may have agreed with Tanaka.

Tanaka's treatment of mental disorders and Reiki's mental treatment both focus on the forehead.

'*Ketsueki Kokan ho*' ('Reiki Finish' or Nerve Stroke) is very similar to Tanaka's finishing technique in treating mental diseases/disorders.

Tanaka emphasizes Reishi should be done with vigor and energy rather than timidly. This was also emphasized in my Reiki training with Sweeney.

Tanaka's treatment calms the patient, and creates tranquility, which also seems to be one of the effects Reiki has on people.

Reiki, like Reishi, is applied one to four times daily as the case requires, but Tanaka mentions some cases should not be applied more than one or two times. Tanaka, Usui-sensei and Hayashi-sensei and Sweeney all seem to correlate on the point that chronic disease may take longer to cure, but that most cases should be resolved within one or two weeks, but with no definitive timeframe as each case is very unique.

The teachings of Taireido, Usui and contemporary Reiki masters are all similar in saying treatment to self or others may balance mind and body and can be a great preventive medicine to all ills.

Tanaka, like Usui and Sweeney speaks much about cures – it may make one wonder if all these similarities are coincidence or if they spring from the same source? The word 'Cure' is fundamental to the teachings of these masters.

There are practices that I have had the privilege to be part of and that I found very familiar when reading the passages concerning treatment methods.

My introduction to Reiki, at the age of 17 years, happened perhaps by chance. I was with a friend at a local 'mind, body, spirit fair.' As we walked past the door of a Danish Reiki Master who was about to hold a session of Group Treatment, we decided to join in. He talked for about 2 minutes on what Reiki was, and gave simple instructions to sit down, relax, breath deep and calm with our eyes closed. Then the session started. It seemed everyone in the room was surprised by the powerful effects. After he opened up for questions from the floor, my friend asked simply what he had done, upon which he replied: 'I just relaxed, meditated, and moved the energy through me and around the room.'

Reading the group treatment as described by Tanaka, it strikes me as too similar for it to be mere coincidence, and seems 'part and parcel' of these therapies potentials.

During my Reiki courses with Allan Sweeney, we stood in a circle holding hands, and he initiated clockwise movement of the energy around the circle, which was distinctly felt by all who partook in the circle. He also explained other versions of this technique. To my surprise, this is exactly how Tanaka explains it. The Reiki world seems embedded with Taireido.

Tanaka's opening remarks about treatment at a distance, or distant/absent treatment concern repetitive skill of students to practice 'Treatment at a distance.' He emphasizes quality of training. His approach to healing and training is methodological, a scientific approach of the day. Usui said he hoped the practice would one day be compatible with science. Sweeney has undertaken various forms of research into cancer, deafness, attention deficit hyperactive disorder, tinnitus, back pain, depression, migraine, fractures and emotions, all of which show significant outcomes. Nowadays science undertakes formal research into Reiki, which shows outstanding therapeutic and/or medical results.

Tanaka focuses on the students' ability to achieve success that can be documented by oral or written comments of patients (qualitative comments on outcomes) and their capacity to achieve high percentages of success that are assessed by a number being reduced over time. For example on a scale of 1-10, pain may be a 9 before Reiki, and only a 3 after, showing 2/3 reduction in pain (quantitative percentages of outcomes). This is exactly how I was presented and taught Reiki by my teacher, Sweeney, and how Reiki is academically researched now. There seems little room for ingenuity – only the ability to repeat the master's techniques as precisely as possible in order to achieve repeatable high success rates. Similarities again…

Persons who use or research Tanaka's 'Distant/Absent Healing' may find that although this section predates Reiki, it is identical even in the wording of the description of the technique as presented by Takata-sensei and Tanaka, to how modern Reiki practitioners practice 'Distant/Absent healing.' This may evidence a strong link between Tanaka and Reiki.

So for example, Takata-sensei taught 'absent healing' identical to Tanaka's 'Treatment at a distance.' Because Takata's teaching came via Hayashi-sensei and Usui-sensei, and are identical to Tanaka's teachings, it seems highly probable that Takata's lineage goes back further to Tanaka.

It should be noted that according to the 'Hikkei', Usui also taught 'remote therapy', which was almost identical in language to how Tanaka described distant therapy – and that Hayashi used this information.

It therefore seems Takata, Hayashi and Usui were familiar with Tanaka's teachings.

Even though most of the written records from Taireido disappeared when their main temple burned down in 1926, it is possible that Tanaka's books were read by Takata-sensei when she arrived in Japan in 1935. Despite the accidental burning of many Taireido documents, many must have existed in private homes and collections. Especially, serious practitioners of the art would have owned their own copy of Taireido. If I, a serious Reiki enthusiast could find four copies of this book, other serious practitioners from 70 or 80 years ago are highly likely also to have found these works. Also, it took me only a few weeks to trace most of the work given out by Tanaka, so it gives a good chance that Usui-sensei, Hayashi-sensei, and Takata-sensei found the teachings too.

Reiki practitioners are often taught 'distant' or 'absent' healing treatment on Reiki II courses. Tanaka does not seem to use the Reiki '*Hon Sha Ze Sho Nen*', but uses a different focusing technique, '*Reiyû*'霊融 (Fusion with the Spirit). Apart from this, the two techniques or methods are identical, in thought, word and action.

> "*Hon Sha Ze Sho Nen*' has taken on many meanings along its journey; commonly it is thought of as an aid to send Reiki through time or space; to connect to someone or something; or to interact with the 'spirit world.' Translation of the '*Jumon*' or Symbol '*Hon Sha Ze Sho Nen*,' may suggest a meaning for the symbol. "Correct Thought/ Mindfulness is the essence of being"[26]
>
> "In some Japanese forms of Reiki (Gendai Reiki ho), Symbol 3 (*Hon Sha Ze Sho Nen*) is seen as representing the transcendent 'oneness' within the practitioner, and the realization that there is no separation between the two people sharing the phenomenon of giving-receiving Reiki.
>
> "In yet other Japanese styles - Hekikuu Reiki for example - *Hon Sha Ze Sho Nen* is taught neither as a 'distant' symbol, nor as a symbol of 'oneness' but rather as one pertaining to mindfulness and the mental faculties in general."
>
> James Deacon[27]

Concepts of transcendence, connection, correct thought or mindfulness are foundations to aid focus. This applies to Reiki symbol use, and preparations of the Reiyû technique in Reishi.

Reiyû (fusion with the spirit) also uses focus and generation of Reishi in the navel area which, combined with the method 'Treatment at a Distance' immediately generates Reishi Action within the receiver.

26-26 James Deacon, http://www.aetw.org/Reiki_symbolsD.html

'Distant Treatment' has led to heated discussions. The ability to transcend Time & Space makes Reiki a time-travelling agent of healing for some; others find transcendence of time and space difficult to accept. This 'conflict' could be explained with the mental construct that Reiki is purely a Newtonian 'energy', moving through space, through us, to the receiver, and having a healing effect. Usui and Tanaka speak of this similarly, naming it both spiritual and physical, so once again, Usui teaches the same as Tanaka.

In the context of Distant Treatment, the Reishi Action/Reiki Action is seen as transcendental – and again the two systems coincide.

Tanaka's ideas on the transcendent aspects of Reishi, and Reishi as a substance of the universe, are similar to ideas of Usui and modern science. Accordingly the teachings of Taireido pertaining to the Reishi Action, or Usui's Reiki the phenomenon is seen to transcend duality; for example physicality and spirituality; energy and matter; time and space. Reishi or Reiki is thus considered the power of God, Universe, or any other terminology used to express universal creative forces.

Reishi Distant Treatment was not so much that energy travelled through space or time as a medium. Rather it transcended them both, hence emphasis that practitioners maintain a transcendent state of mind giving immediate effect over distance. These points may be compatible. Energy may travel through space or time with immediate effect, as accepted in modern physics.

Non-locality is the ability of an object to directly influence another distant object, termed in quantum physics as entanglement. Tanaka said the practitioner generates Reishi Action in another being to effect a treatment by maintaining a connection through transcendent aspect of Reishi. This could be achieved through the non-locality aspect of this force. These thoughts are also expressed amongst many modern Reiki practitioners, who by personal experience or through methods of teaching, are under the impression that one triggers the Reiki phenomena in the other person, which in turn has the healing effect. These practitioners see themselves mostly as facilitators of the effect, not that it is something that passes through them. Again, Tanaka and many modern masters agree with each other.

Tanaka states that patients may be unaware of treatment and emphasizes that recovery rate is highly important, and not sensations the treatment may give. Tanaka emphasizes that one should focus on the person to be treated, and be familiarized with a patient's ailment. Greater focus gives greater outcome. An echo found in modern Reiki practice, where the focus is on dedicated effort, and not to get attached to the sensations that might occur. Chapter 9 in Sweeney's book, 'The Reiki 1 Manual' also explains this.

Tanaka says distant treatment time is not more than 5 minutes and treatment method is the same for all types of illness. Focus is on one patient's ailment and treatment at a time. This is taught by Sweeney, although other modern methods give distant treatment to a list of people at the same time. Logically, modern methods may not be as effective as an individual focused treatment, because each individual may have different needs?

Tanaka said the main point to achieve success is Self-Transcendence, key to most teachings in Taireido. Similarly I was taught to practice self-transcendence in Reiki as the core of every Reiki practice, by connecting to a greater Reiki source, and turn Reiki-On. It is not meditation, rather a self-transcendent knowing.

Whatever triggers the healing response in the patient is not as important as the fact that there are improvements in the patient's condition. However, Tanaka's sentiment here seems familiar to some Reiki practitioners who feel that there is no transference of energy per se but rather a facilitation to awaken the inherent Reiki (healing force) within the patient. Nonetheless it is still Reiki or Reishi that is the cause of the healing effect whether by transmission or by trigger effect, and honestly I feel that both founders were aware of this dual nature of the Reiki or Reishi, and explored these aspects in their methods.

Takata-sensei, in her own words, reminds us that the patient is not an inactive participant in this process. This is because, even though the Reiki like the Reishi Action will have effect whether the patient is aware or not, an active patient will benefit their own healing process. Tanaka himself noticed this, especially with patients requesting distant treatments.

> "The patient who is about to receive this treatment must purify one's thoughts, feel comfortable, and a desire to get well. One must not forget to feel grateful. Gratitude is a great cure for the mind..."
>
> *Takata-sensei*[28]

[28] James Deacon, http://www.aetw.org/Reiki_takata_taught.htm

TAIREIDO, REISHI & REIKI

The Spiritual aspect of Taireido is self evident throughout this work. Morihei Tanaka puts a lot of emphasis on the importance of understanding and comprehension of this aspect in the practical application of 'The Science of Reishi' or as he also calls it 'reiri gaku' The whole system of thought known as Taireido, and the art and science of Reishi is based on Tanaka's enlightenment.

The story of Tanaka studying the various religious doctrines of the world, and practicing rigid spiritual discipline whilst alone in the mountains of his village, close to Kyoto, is identical to the story we are told of the founder of Reiki, Mikao Usui. The method and the results, of discovering the therapeutic properties of this experience or phenomena is the same, also the story of both founders discovering, almost by chance, the effects this had on others upon their return down the mountain. Upon returning from the mountain, both founders apparently healed a young girl of toothache.

Tanaka sets out to outline his understanding of his satori or kantoku experience. Naming his understanding of the ultimate source of all that is as 'TAIREI', or 'The Great Spirit', 'TAIREIDO' could be understood as "the way of the Great Spirit". The study of 'TAIREIDO' is called 'Reiri-gaku', and would include both the theoretical and the practical aspects.

'REISHI', the active power or force emanating from the source was the basis for all that is, and Tanaka coined the term 'Reishi' for this 'God-power'. Now this is too close to brush off as a coincidence when looking at the teachings of Usui Reiki Ryoho. We are taught that Reiki is the ultimate source of all that is, we are also told that Reiki is the active force or power of this source.

This understanding of the teachings that have come to us from Usui-sensei, is that Reiki refers to both something spiritual and Divine, and at the same time to the active ingredient often called 'Life-force' or 'Ki', 'Qi/Chi' or 'prana'.

Reiki is often read broken up into its component kanji, as well as its meaning as a kanji pair. Rei and Ki, often understood as spirit or spiritual (rei) life-force (ki). However it is also possible to read the 'ki' kanji as only referring to the active element of Rei, f.eks. Spirit/Spiritual-force, Spirit/ Spiritual-action.

Now if this was done to 'Reishi,' one might lose a bit of its true meaning. Reishi can be translated to spirit/spiritual-strength or spirit/spiritual-force. If broken up it can be read as Spirit/Soul (rei), and child (shi), and could be read as spirit-child, or even ghost-child. These comments are simply trying to highlight translation and transliteration from Japanese to English, and are only meant to be suggestions on which readers can make up their own minds.

The part of the work that puts forth the spiritual doctrine of Taireido, as understood and formulated by Moriehei Tanaka, may also be found in the spiritual teachings of Reiki. The words used by the founders of these two systems clearly show that they must have had similar thoughts as well as vocabulary to express these ideas so identically. In both systems, the spiritual path seemed to be overshadowed by the therapeutic, and the emphasis is on treatment of disease. Yet, both these systems hold that they are first and foremost a spiritual path - treatment of disease is integrated into the spiritual path, and the Spirit is put as the reason for the healing to happen.

Depending on how these two systems are approached by modern practitioners, they can focus either on a spiritual path, or a healing path, or an integration of the two. Both Tanaka and Usui-sensei seem to have promoted their systems as spiritual healing systems, and at the same time recognized the physical healing that takes place through Ki and Light as well as through the spiritual power of Reishi/Tairei or Reiki

In Reiki practice, we speak of: Reiki, the system; Reiki, the healing force or energy; Reiki as the source. In dissecting the meanings put to each concept, we might be able to see how Tairei and Reishi fits with the concepts in Reiki.

Takata-sensei explained Reiki as: 'a universal force from the Great Divine Spirit' - we could easily read this as: 'Reiki is a universal force from Tairei.'

She also called it 'God Power', similarly Tanaka does the same in relating the relationship between Reishi and Tairei: 'The universe is product of one all-pervading principle called REISHI, which is an emanation of TAIREI and the means by which the latter manifests itself in creation.' In this context Reiki and Reishi are very much interchangeable.

Takata-sensei explains more what Reiki is: 'It is not associated with any visible material being.' 'It is an unseen spiritual power that radiates vibration and lifts one into harmony. This power is incomprehensible to man, yet every single living being is receiving its blessings...'[29]

Again we can see striking similarities when comparing it to Tanaka's explanations: 'The Light and Power of TAIREI are eternal and omnipresent, the primal source of existence from which the world draws all sustenance.'

Considering that both Tanaka and Usui, among others, were considered to have 'reijutsu' (spiritual powers or spiritual skill) and Tanaka called the source of this power, simply, the Great Spirit just like Takata did in trying to explain Reiki. This reasoning if extended, seems that we could consider Dai Kô Myô, or the Rei in Reiki as Usui-sensei's reference to the source of this power. Tanaka goes to great lengths in explaining his enlightenment and discovery of these spiritual principals as we can see here:

> 'Reishi is the active principle of TAIREI, the Great Spirit. It is the process by which the Divine life and power work'
>
> 'A knowledge of Reishi is how to use a power within you, of which TAIREI is the origin'
>
> 'Reishi is the source of all life: in it the fusing of the spiritual and material becomes real.'

Similarly to Reiki, is the Science of Reishi, in that there is no specific mental training required, and proficiency in the Art can be achieved in a very short time, and does not take years of mental training. This is very unique to Reiki and Tanaka's Science of Reishi. Sweeney also teaches that cures can be obtained in a short time with the right knowledge.

> "Mental abstraction is not forbidden as a method of mental culture, but it is not to be attempted in connection with Reishi. The external action of Reishi has no connection with cultivation of mind; and as the external action of Reishi is due to oneself any occupation of the mind with other matters must necessarily hinder it."

In relation to bodily attitude, Tanaka, similar to my Reiki training with Sweeney, states categorically 'When the posture is inaccurate, or causes any unnatural physical strain, the realization of the action of Reishi is prevented.'

---

29 Takata Diaries 1935/1936, http://www.aetw.org/Reiki_takata_diary.htm

The skills developed in the Reiki and Reishi system are natural skills that everyone possesses. This is an idea that is carried in both systems of thought and the ease of learning these skills or gaining these powers is very simple and easy. As we will see in this volume, Tanaka provides the same answer as we can find in what is reputed to be Usui's writings.

> "Even those at the beginning of their initiation have been able impressively to exercise the spiritual powers of healing. If you care to think of it, it will seem incomprehensible that within a little time one can be endowed with the spiritual power to cure a disease, which is considered the most difficult task a person can undertake. I think that is an extremely natural reaction. However, the ability to accomplish this most difficult task with ease is the special feature of our spiritual therapy"
>
> Mikao Usui, Reiki Hikkei[30]

Contemporary Reiki history has many different claims of "original teachings." Some seem reasonable, others seem like wild imagination. Today we may finally be able to shed some light on the true roots of the Reiki system, providing real documentation and clear historical references, and thus, finally ending the hearsay and assumptive arguments regarding the "true" roots and teachings of Mikao Usui. We hope this work will enlighten the reader, and clearly show how closely the system of thought developed and promoted by Morihei Tanaka, TAIREIDO and the Science of Reishi, resembles the system of Mikao Usui, Usui Reiki Ryoho.

We hope that this work will encourage further study in the field by reputable Reiki-History researchers.

Frank Shortt

---

[30] Dr. Allan Sweeney "Explanation of Reiki Therapy" © 1998, and "The Reiki 1 Manual" © 2002

INTRODUCTION

By Allan Sweeney

Trying to make sense of history

Reiki masters have often discussed the origins of Reiki, and even more often debated what knowledge should be taught. Sometimes discussions and debates are due to scant available written documentation from Dr Usui, Dr Hayashi, and Mrs Takata, who made Reiki most known in the world.

Peculiarly, the more recent the Reiki history from those important figures, the less writings there were. Or, put another way, the further back in time you go, the more writings are available.

1. 40 years ago in the 1970s, Mrs Takata wrote no manuals at all, and did not let students write notes of courses.
2. 90 years ago approx. in the 1920s, Dr Usui wrote about Reiki as a therapy. Usui was reputed to give students notes and manuals.

This book describes another historical figure.

3. 100 years ago approx., in the 1910s, years before Dr Usui's first writings, the man often recognised as Dr Usui's teacher, Morihei Tanaka, wrote several full books explaining his Taireido therapy. These volumes contained extensive, in-depth knowledge of how healing and spirituality could help Mankind. This book will describe these writings and how they relate to Dr Usui's writings and philosophy, through to Takata and modern-day masters.

Yet even though 1910s and 1920s writings give knowledge on healing as a therapy, or on possible origins and teachings of Reiki, it was how Mrs Takata taught in the 1970s that helped Reiki spread around the world to become a global brand.

Lineages

In the Reiki world, a big deal is made about 'lineage.' Masters ask, 'Who was a student's teacher, who was their teacher's teacher', and so on etc, with a lineage going back to Usui.

Most lineages however have become undervalued, because most people in most lineages will just teach their own way anyway. A particular lineage is little guarantee of quality. In some cases, a lineage can even be a guarantee of bad quality.

Nowadays, almost regardless of who someone's teacher is, no-one knows who teaches what and how. It has got to the stage where some in government, academic and medical establishments frown on Reiki as a repeatable therapy, because they cannot be sure what they will get for their money.

Some hospitals and surgeries employ Reiki therapists, but employment is usually on a local basis. Those in authority, who question the validity of what type of Reiki a therapist will give, seem to be increasing. A lineage has little meaning for them – they are more interested in the professional quality of the individual practitioner.

Even grassroots populations seem to be wondering or doubtful of the type or Reiki out there. A lineage has little meaning also to them – rather, they need to know how effective a particular therapist's outcomes are for their particular condition.

Maybe it's time to look at the roots of Reiki as a healing therapy. Looking back into the past might even improve Reiki in the future as a therapy for goodness – and that could be a blessing for us all.

1970s Mrs Takata's 'Traditional Usui Reiki'

Mrs Takata should be honored big-time for her role in spreading Reiki around the world. Without her, Reiki probably would not be the global force for goodness it is now.

But it's important to be realistic too. According to Barbara Ray, Mrs Takata chose not to teach knowledge she'd gained in Japan. Instead she gave attunements, and much time for students to practice giving each other Reiki therapy. That's based on stories from students who studied with her.

In 1938 Takata-sensei had learned Reiki from Dr Hayashi, who had studied with Usui-sensei. 32 years later, in 1970, Takata began teaching Reiki. It is unlikely that something studied 32 years previously could be taught perfectly. But because Takata said she was the only living Reiki master, her teachings were respected as being 'Traditional Usui Reiki.'

This is not meant to denigrate Takata-sensei as she did a great job, but one of the problems with Reiki as a therapy was that there was little 'traditional' or of 'Usui' in Takata's teachings because she didn't teach much knowledge. So her students and their students around the world who said they taught 'Traditional Usui Reiki' actually didn't. Perhaps their teachings could have been called 'Traditional **Takata** Reiki.'

But during the 1970s and 1980s, there was no other well known source of knowledge about Dr Usui or traditional Reiki. The only well known knowledge on Reiki, was whatever Takata told. So no-one questioned her, and countless masters called their teachings 'Traditional Usui Reiki', not knowing they were actually using 'Traditional **Takata** Reiki.'

As mentioned, 'Traditional Takata Reiki' was founded on giving students an attunement, to enable natural development as Reiki healers. Students then practiced sharing Reiki healing with each other, for much of the course time, and self-learning from personal therapy experiences.

Takata had no in-depth manual, and mainly did not allow her teachings to be written down, although little actual teaching or knowledge was imparted to students. Because Mrs Takata taught little on her classes, and her 22 students had no syllabus for teaching knowledge, they all taught whatever they wanted. And all the students of Takata's 22 masters also taught whatever they wanted too, so did their students, and so on.

So by the time Reiki spread via Takata around the world, millions of teachers, in every country on Earth, could more or less teach whatever they wanted to teach.

Which is why nowadays you can learn Reiki is almost anything. I've seen 'Angel Reiki', 'Massage Reiki', 'Reiki and Aliens', 'Naked Reiki' and so on. Almost any mystical subject could come under the Reiki umbrella somewhere from some master. No-one knows exactly what they'll get nowadays when they go to a Reiki therapist or teacher.

1920s Dr Usui's true 'Traditional Usui Reiki'

Usui's writings included a description of how Reiki came to him, his beliefs, spiritual therapy, and how Reiki could help specific conditions. Dr Usui also describes how Reiki was debated in the Japanese parliament, with quotes from doctors in the Japan Medical Bulletin, and hopes for future compatibility with science.

In particular, Dr Usui's writings showed that Reiki was first and foremost a therapy to heal self, family and patients – he used the word 'cure' many times. Allan Sweeney's 504-page book, "The Reiki 1 Manual incorporating the Spiritual Healer's Guide" includes Usui-sensei's writings and full commentaries. Dr Usui is shown to be enthusiastic, spiritual, tough, dedicated, and professional in his approach as a healer and teacher, and in his work and hopes with government, doctors and scientists.

It was known that Dr Usui sought teachings for many years from others. Yet exactly whose teachings and what teachings have remained largely speculation. The one name that regularly crops up as being the teacher of Dr Usui is Morihei Tanaka.

1910s Morihei Tanaka's 'Taireido'

This volume, written in English, is a collection from Tanaka's previous volumes published in Japan in 1910 and 1916. It is quite apparent Dr Usui used at least some of the teachings from Tanaka's books because some of the language is identical. Also, their spiritual philosophy and the lists of treatable conditions are very similar. The main question may be: did some of Usui-sensei's knowledge come directly from studying with Tanaka, or indirectly from reading Tanaka's many publications.

Dr Usui's Society

I regret feeling the need to write this paragraph, but some Reiki masters suggest Usui's Society still exists, and tries to control Reiki. A search of the internet shows websites that make various allegations against Usui's Society. Certainly the Society does not seem to have published substantial books or materials to benefit Mankind. Certain of their teachers are alleged to openly make accusations against other Reiki masters, and offer little to heal rifts. If the internet is true, certain of the Usui Society's teachers may soon seek ways even to put down this book. These allegations and negative potentials may not be true – but wait and see...

Future Reiki research focus

It may be interesting for research-focused readers of this book to move back in their Reiki research before Takata, before Usui, and before Usui's Society – as little is known from original writings of any of them. Instead, perhaps it's time to adequately explore the writings of Morihei Tanaka, and then potentially honour him as the teacher of Usui, and the forerunner for Usui's organisation.

Summary

To summarize, many problems with Reiki history are due to the lack of extensive original historical writings from important sources such as Takata, Usui, and Usui's Society. There is a large gap in the knowledge of Reiki as a healing therapy, and its history. It is hoped that this book on Taireido by Tanaka, who is often suggested as the teacher of Dr Usui, can go some way to fill that gap. The therapies, methods and philosophies of Taireido may at last give substantial evidence that Reiki could be based more on spirituality, health improvement, and on relieving the suffering of Mankind.

Some people say that history is not too relevant, that it's the 'now' that's most important. However, if by bringing these historical issues into the open, perhaps an understanding of the past of Reiki that was steeped in spirituality, cures, and research processes, can only be a blessing. Because then true truth might be unveiled to make sense of Reiki as its founders intended – a loving spiritual and healing system founded on scientific research. It would probably honor Tanaka and Usui for modern practitioners to academically research techniques that, compared to other therapies are quicker, easier, more effective, less dangerous, cheaper to provide, more repeatable – and provide more permanent outcomes. And then perhaps the past may lead to stepping stones towards an even more harmonious and loving Reiki future.

Allan Sweeney

TAIREIDO
A NEW REVELATION THE SPIRITUAL, MENTAL AND PHYSICAL SALVATION OF MANKIND

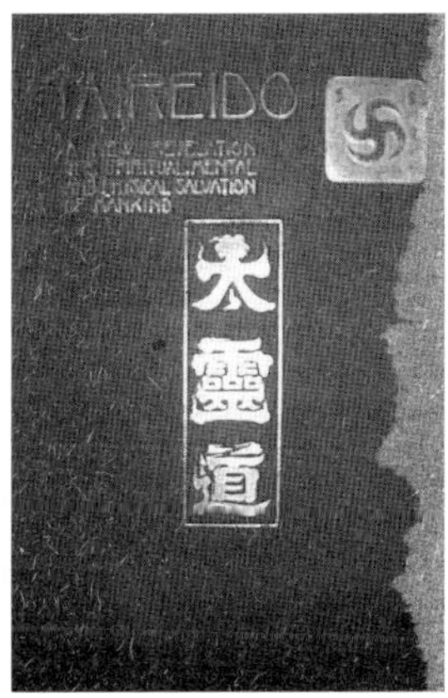

TAIREIDO: A NEW REVELATION FOR THE SPIRITUAL, MENTAL AND PHYSICAL SALVATION OF MANKIND

By

TANAKA MORIHEI
FOUNDER OF TAIREIDO

TAIREIDO HONIN 1920

PRINTED
By
THE JAPAN MAGAZINE CO.
Tokyo, Japan

EDITED BY
Frank Shortt & Allan Sweeney
(2009 - 2010)

PREFACE

Man has reached the most crucial period in his history. The whole world is calling for reconstruction and no one appears able to undertake the task. Religion, Philosophy, Science and Socialism have failed and League of Nations is not yet consummated. The war between classes, the strong against the weak, menaces the very existence of civilization. How are justice and righteousness to be evolved out of the present contradiction and chaos? The change can come in only one way: by diverting the human mind from material to spiritual considerations, the utilization of all material power for spiritual ends. Man has in him the Power to do this if he will but learn how to exert it. He must seek spiritual rather than material expansion. Man's soul is immortal; and Man's hope is in himself. The body cannot be healthy or free if the soul is in slavery to material things.

The era of soul dominance is here; but the world has not begun to realize the meaning of human existence. For the reconstruction of the world and the remaking of man I offer TAIREIDO, a new system of life revealed to me after years of contemplation and divine communion.

TAIREIDO reveals to man the inherent Power with which Heaven has endowed him for the perfect regulation of the world of life and civilization. Once man acquires knowledge of this system and acquires the art of Reishi he has mastered the secrets of existence, and commands the power and wisdom to live a rational life unhindered by the disturbing and irregular forces of evil. In TAIREIDO lies the power to overthrow materialism and bring about a civilization based on soul qualities. By TAIREIDO a man becomes able to express the divinity within him, letting it shine forth in glowing radiance upon the world. A careful perusal of the following pages will indicate in some measure how this is true.

TANAKA MORIHEI

Founder of Taireido

Tokyo, 1920

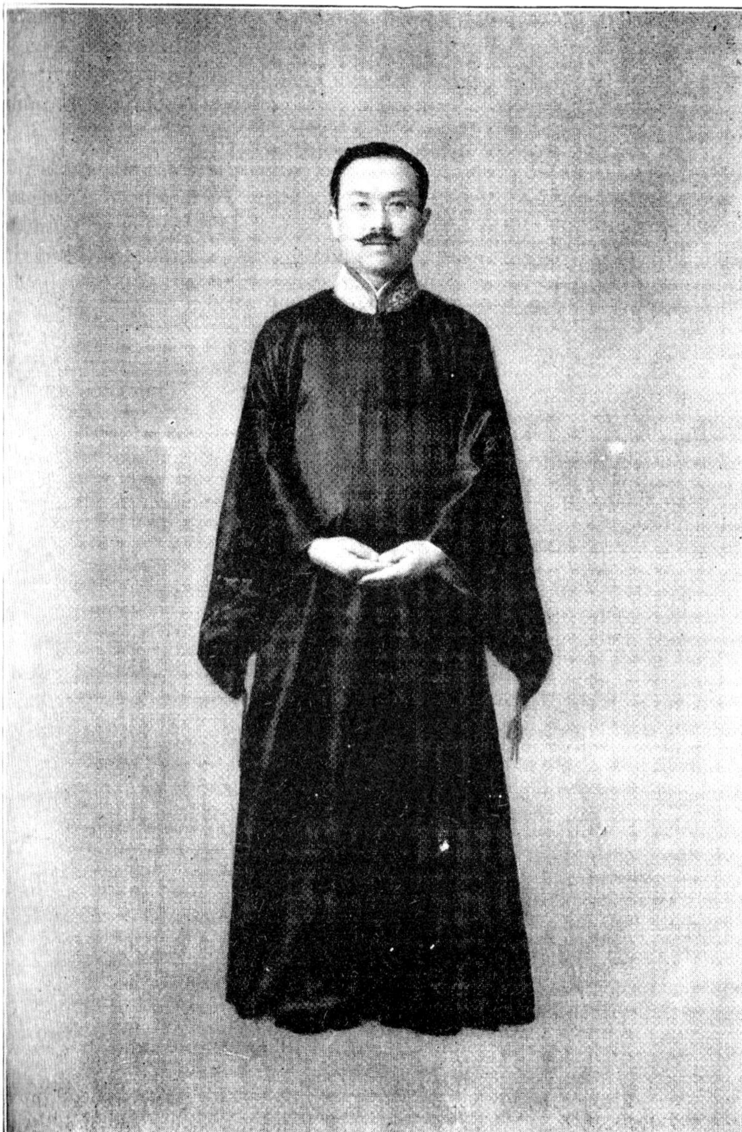

Correct Position
TANAKA MORIHEI

A FOREWORD

WHAT IS TAIREIDO

1. The Greatest Good[31]

The Supreme Purpose of TAIREIDO[32] is to unify human thought and life so as to bring about security of mind and perfect physical condition. By this reconstruction of human life, mentally and physically, a perfect world will be constituted. Contemporary thought drifts among spiritualism, materialism and atheism, finding no goal or rest. The human mind at present is adrift upon a sea of darkness. Few understand the significance of human life, see even any value in it, and thus remain ignorant of mans' true destiny. There is no central truth that commands universal loyalty. Men labor in pursuit of wealth or fame, indifferent to the real object and value of this life. Human life as it appears today is a sad scene of doubt and uncertainty. How irrational it is for man to go on acting thus blindly, unconscious of the significance and value of the life he lives!

Every self-conscious human being is able to assure themselves of the reality of human life. Once persuaded of the reality of life how can any rational person go on living as if fame and power and wealth were all! Yet is not this the only substance in the lives of most people today? It seems as if it were not given to many people in the world to realize more than this vain sort of existence. At least such is the impression one gets of contemporary society. Now what is it that man needs to change all this and bring him to the goal of true existence? It is true thought! It is for want of true thought that contemporary life is so restless and most souls as lonely as wanderers in the desert. TAIREIDO has been revealed to man to form a centre of thought round which all minds may rally and which all minds may serve, to find life. It is the Light of the world summoning the lost and wandering to the haven of true existence. Everyone who follows this Light will be free from the present mental and spiritual desolation that most men feel. The mind will be secure and peaceful, within the grasp of universal thought.

---

[31] This opening paragraph uses powerful words for any society at any time

[32] Throughout the book, Tanaka writes TAIREIDO in capital letters

2. TAIREIDO Comprehends yet Transcends Philosophy, Ethics and Religion

Through the ages Religion has persisted and developed as a necessary demand of the human mind. Man has felt that Religion was essential to the unity of his thought and the security of his mind. But contemporary thought cannot be freed from confusion and unified, so as to bring man satisfaction and peace, simply by praying to the God of the Christians or the Amida of the Buddhist. The power of religion is belief or faith. Without this belief there is no communion with the God of the Christians or the Amida of the Buddhist[33]. Now before belief can come there must be understanding. It is maintained that God and Amida transcend reason; but if the mind is expected to believe without understanding the reason of the transcendence or reason, the result is mere credulity or superstition. In this way there can be no true ground of belief. TAIREIDO does not ask men to believe. It simply reveals itself to them as the Substance of all things in a way that their understanding can grasp and utilize. When the mind apprehends and uses a thing there is no difficulty in believing in it[34]. The understanding compels the will to believe. How TAIREIDO may be understood and used by all men is fully explained in the body of this work.

If the various chapters of this volume are carefully perused and acted upon there will be a full understanding of TAIREIDO, the Substance of the Universe, on which all mind and matter depend. The first part of the volume deals with the nature of TAIREIDO and how one can apprehend it. Every word of this book is true and charged with Truth's inspiration. Once the student has thoroughly digested the principles herein laid down, and acts upon them, he will have no difficulty in understanding how the Universal Essence transcends while including all the truth of Religion. It is therefore, superior to religion while giving religion its validity. Only the man who apprehends the reality and significance of TAIREIDO can fully appreciate the meaning of religion.

Some cannot accept Religion but allow Ethics. In the past ethics has been at times associated with religion and at times divorced there from. Generally, however, religion has concerned itself with belief in God or Buddha, while ethics has laid down the fundamentals of morality as a standard of life. As age increases it becomes easier to fall into line with traditional ethics, which are chiefly of a negative nature and require no more than submission. The

---

[33] Tanaka understood diverse religions on which to base his system

[34] Usui argues the same in the '*Hikkei*'

Oriental ethics based on family life and the Western ethics based on individualism differ somewhat in regard to what is esteemed good and bad; so that sometimes what is considered bad in the West is not considered so in the East, and vice versa. As internationalism expands the world will be thus more confused than ever, and unity of thought be still further hindered. The standards of morality must be of universal import and appeal. Until this is so the mind of man will wander and be lost. TAIREIDO does not concern itself with such questions as good and bad: it reveals the perfect truth of life, and thus all darkness and doubt are dispelled. A prior question to the goodness or badness of an action is as to whether the action is based on TRUTH. If it be the outcome of TRUTH it will be a perfect action. Moral standards have always differed according to time and circumstance. But the principles of TAIREIDO have been eternally true. They did not arise from racial geography or outcome but inhere eternally in the nature of existence. The principles of TAIREIDO, as laid down in this volume, give the essentials of TRUTH, and so of LIFE. They have nothing to do with negation or more submission. There are no "Don'ts" in the TAIREIDO creed. TAIREIDO is concerned only with what is positive and living: with what man should do rather than with what he should not do. This involves the most progressive of ethical standards, superseding the past and revealing the way for the present and the future. TAIREIDO sets the standard of mental and physical conduct for all human beings, and reveals an eternal morality. It indeed transcends the old ethics as much as the old religion.

Philosophy also has demanded submission from the human mind, claiming to set forth the essential principles of the universe; and both religion and ethics are usually in some degree types of philosophy. At any rate philosophy is at the basis of both religion and ethics. Man may be regarded a philosophical being, and both religion and ethics are natural to him. Philosophy thus possesses the key to life's solution. But the philosophy of the past has contributed little or nothing to the solution of life's mystery; certainly it has added nothing of any great value to Man's thinking and Man's life here. It has been mainly theoretical rather than practical or of active service to man. Philosophy is indeed one of the imperfect sciences. TAIREIDO, on the other hand, gives man all the philosophy of life he either needs or understands. It reveals to man the Eternal Essence whence all Truth comes and by which life lives. Compared with this profound privilege philosophy is as nothing. Those portions of this volume dealing with TAIREIDO in relation to the Universe, the Community, the State, the Individual, as well as with the General Significance of Life, the Fundamental Question, Life and Death, the Complete Self and Eternal Life, all show that TAIREIDO transcends philosophy beyond all question of magnitude. TAIREIDO is the most systematic and complete philosophy yet revealed to man. It settles all questions of the Universe and of man in relation thereto. It lays down the fundamental principles of all existence and all thought. TAIREIDO lends to philosophy any validity it may possess as an appeal to the human mind.

Thus TAIREIDO includes while transcending Religion, Ethics, Philosophy and all systems of thought yet known to man. The essence of all religion, the fundamentals of all morality, and the basis of all philosophy are clearly defined in the principles of TAIREIDO, while this system of thought and life supremely transcends all.

3. The Light of Time

Man cannot live by bread alone: he lives in his thought. Those without true thought are dead or mere puppets. Neither religion nor morality nor philosophy has taught men to think and live aright. Since TAIREIDO includes in itself the essence of all religion, morality and philosophy it gives the world what it most needs; and without TAIREIDO human life can never come to its proper consummation. Those who cannot believe in religion or are doubtful of modern morality and skeptical of the confused or conflicting philosophies that cry aloud, will have no difficulty in believing in TAIREIDO: it is as evident as the sun in the heavens! Once TAIREIDO is studied and apprehended the meaning of Man's life at last becomes plain, his thought is unified and he has permanent peace of mind.

> We believe that the universe is the product of one principle called *Reishi* which is an emanation of *Tairei* true and good[35].

[35] Much in these first pages would be agreed by most modern Reiki masters

IMPORTANT CONSIDERATIONS IN THE TREATMENT OF DISEASES

1. Preparation for Treatment

In order successfully to apply the Internal Action of Reishi to the cure of disease in others the practitioner requires certain careful preparation of mind and body. As the Action transcends all mental and physical action it is important that the mind and body should not interfere, though incomplete control of mental and physical action cannot wholly interfere with transcendent action.[36] This may be seen from the following experiment. If while the patient and the agent are sleeping a third party lifts the hand of the agent and applies the palm to the affected part of the patient the Action of Reishi will be transmitted and the patient experience a cure,[37] both agent and patient at the moment being unconscious of what has taken place. The effect is not quite so perfect, however, or so easy, as in the regular way, especially in the cases of serious diseases. But the result is sufficient to prove how far the Action of Reishi transcends mentality and physiological conditions generally. It is clear that the effect comes through the hand, or any other part of the body practiced in it: and that no such result can be produced by mere mental or physical action or force. This being true, it might too readily be assumed that no mental or physical preparation was necessary in the treatment of disease in others. But if the practitioner desires to be wholly successful the directions with regard to mental and physical preparation should be followed.

It may be difficult for the practitioner to free the mind from ideas associated with ordinary medical treatment and practice, which is based on considerations purely material. He is apt to think of medicine and apparatus and so on: or if not, to suppose that at least mental intention is important. But in Reishi treatment the effect is produced not by mind or by body but by Reishi, the essence or basal force of life, and not by any material force or means. The practitioner has constantly to keep this in mind. He must believe that, as he is in command of this mysterious power, he has absolute dignity and supreme authority over disease, and, therefore so applies the Action of

[36] As is also taught on most Reiki courses today.

[37] This phenomena is often referred to as the 'intelligent nature of Reiki'

Reishi. To reach so high a degree of assurance and personal confidence the practitioner needs preparation[38].

2. The Mental Preparation Most Necessary

For applying successfully the Internal Action of Reishi to the curing of disease in others the following mental virtues must be assiduously cultivated: Transcendence, Solemnity, Conviction, Sympathy, Earnestness, Prudence, Accuracy, Promptitude, Boldness, Impartiality and Tenacity[39].

Transcendence

In speaking of TAIREIDO the word transcendence implies the most profound significance of any in the category of words. To understand transcendence, to hold it and keep it, is the first principle of advancement in the Art of Reishi. This is especially true in regard to effective application of the Art of Reishi to the treatment of disease. When the mind is lost in completely transcendent attitude the agent becomes fully qualified for progress in the Art. To be incapable of this attitude of transcendence is to be disqualified for a practitioner in the Art of Reishi.

In the treatment of disease the practitioner must not be easily discouraged or put off by interference or opposition on the part of the patient or of the patient, or by the nurse, or the sarcasm of unbelievers[40]. These trifles need cost him no thought. His attitude or state of transcendence should also lift him above doubts as to the possibility of healing the disease. He must always be prepared to reach the transcendent state and to do his best to accomplish the healing process; and he can do his best only when he exercises his capacity to transmit the Internal Action of Reishi to the fullest extent. Let the practitioner realize that he himself, who is in possession of Reishi, is of the same body as the patient. In the Art of healing he must know that two divine things have come into contact, and the action of healing is a divine action. Therefore he must be firm as a rock. Nothing of his environment must be allowed to interrupt his action. The Art must be applied in full accordance with the principles of unity a harmony involved in TAIREI.

---

[38] Well-argued, suggesting therapists prepare adequately before treatment

[39] A list of 11 virtues for Tanaka's students to attain. Usui's Hikkei gave a list of virtues such as outstanding results, deporting well and enthusiasm

[40] Usui said in the Hikkei, 'We practitioners of the Usui Reiki Therapy do not mind how much our practices are doubted, held in contempt or rejected.'

Solemnity

The practitioner should also be able to assume a state of profound solemnity, which is necessary to induce in great power the presence of TAIREI and to enable the agent to apply the consequent Action of Reishi to the elimination of disease. The trick of quacks and the jokes of doctors are no use in applying the Action of Reishi. Without due solemnity on part of the practitioner either he or the patient may not treat the Action with proper care, for it must be understood that carelessness always lessens efficacy. All talk or conversation between agent and the patient is strictly forbidden. Servant or others present must likewise observe silence. It is, however, all right for the practitioner to inquire, when necessary, as to the painfulness or other effect of any operation executed by the practitioner. But only questions absolutely essential to proper treatment should be asked[41]. The agent should never indulge in tobacco either before, during or immediately after performing treatment. Nor must anyone in the room be allowed to use tobacco. If necessary the practitioner may speak to enforce this rule. The agent must not be under the influence of alcohol in any form, and must refrain from applying the Action of Reishi to any patient under such influence. The Art should not be practiced in any room save one specially prepared for the operation. No witnesses should be permitted, save nurses or attendants that may be necessary. Solemnity should pervade all. Mere affected solemnity won't do. Thus with an environment of profound solemnity the practitioner is able to keep proper solemnity and with a free mind can apply the Art of Reishi.

Sincerity

It seems hardly necessary to remind the student that nothing can be accomplished without sincerity. To be otherwise than serious in the treatment of human affliction is unpardonable. Often illness is a matter of life and death. Sincerity is essential to leaving a proper impression on the patient as well as to be effective agent of the transmission of the Action of Reishi. Without sincerity the practitioner cannot make the necessary preparations here outlined. If the practitioner be insincere toward the patient he will be likewise toward the Art of Reishi; and *vice versa*.

---

[41] The previous 3 sentences are taught in modern systems e.g. Sweeney's

Conviction

When it is said that conviction is essential to the successful practice of the Art of Reishi it is not meant that Reishi may be dependent on mental or physical conditions, for the effectiveness of the Action of Reishi is not so dependent. The proper application of the Art of Reishi, however, depends much on whether the practitioner is convicted in the theory and practice that the mysterious power of Reishi can heal diseases. To attempt to apply to others what one does not believe in oneself is unworthy of any man. One cannot expect others to treat with respect what one is not convinced of oneself. The conviction insisted on here is not a kind of faith, such as religion speaks of: it is a full understanding of the reality of Reishi as an Art of divine power for the removal of disease. It is simply the conviction of one who knows. Belief without knowledge will not render an agent successful in the practice of the Art of Reishi; and any attempt to substitute superstitious faith for conviction completely disqualifies one for practicing Reishi. Once truly convinced in theory and practice that the principles of Reishi are true, and true independently of his either liking or fact, or believing in it, the practitioner can go on and practice the Art. It is a matter in which faith and understanding go together. With proper conviction the agent is prepared to practice the Art and to fight for it, fearing not to face the world. Only with such conviction can one hope to exhibit at all times the authority which TAIREIDO gives, and thus render the Action of Reishi effective.

Sympathy

Sympathy is a human virtue possible to all, and one most essential in the treatment of disease. Existing medical science, being based on materialistic conceptions, has, as a rule, little sympathy with suffering humanity, taking disease as a matter of course. The constant contact with illness, and the unchanging round of prescription for each kind of bodily affection, renders the action purely mechanical, until the physician becomes accustomed to witnessing pain that he feels no special sympathy with the patient. This, perhaps, may be unavoidable, but it is nevertheless regrettable. There is no doubt that the most sympathetic physician will be the best qualified for success, other things being equal. No one will employ a physician if convinced of lack of sympathy on the part of the professional man. And no student of medicine can make proper progress and completely equip themselves for treatment of human disease without some modicum of sympathy. In the application of the Art of Reishi genuine sympathy with those who are to be treated is absolutely necessary. In practicing the Art of

Reishi the agent is wholly under its influence: it controls his spirit, mind and body: all of which makes true sympathy an important factor in success.

Earnestness

When earnestness is advocated as a condition of successful application of the Action of Reishi, undue zeal bordering on frenzy or mania is not meant; but simply the common earnestness that is essential to any kind of success. The overzealous are often as ineffective as those without zeal. The External and Internal Action of Reishi should both be practiced with the utmost earnestness and devotion, but with no excitement and unusual ardor. When the agent is so vitally and enthusiastically given to the practice of the Art that he is consumed by it, he is too earnest and will lose the transcendent state necessary to effective exercise of the Art. In applying the Art of Reishi to disease the agent must naturally be profoundly earnest, but not to the point of refusing to allow the state of transcendence. He must be in earnest about it but not crazy about it. The state of transcendence must be assured so as to transmit the Internal Action of Reishi quite effectively. If the practitioner attempts to apply the Art with cool indifference the result of the mysterious Art will prove less efficacious.

Prudence

In practicing the Art of Reishi prudence is the mother of solemnity; and so care in this respect preserves both virtues. It is by prudence that one examines carefully into the ailment and follows up the results of treatment and the general progress of the case[42]. Even the regular physician has to examine his patient daily and try to reach a correct diagnosis. Any degree of carelessness or undue haste in examination exposes the patient to suffering and suspicion. Want of prudence and care often brings misfortune to a patient. In the application of Reishi to the cure of disease the greatest care must be taken to secure correct knowledge of the case and prudently apply the treatment. In fact no effort of human being requires more prudence, seeing that a human life is entrusted to the care of another. The agent must, therefore, exercise the greatest prudence and apply his Art to the best of his ability, discharging his duties effectively. It is a matter of the most supreme importance to act up to one's responsibility in this respect.

[42] Shows Tanaka was 'academic,' advocating keeping adequate records

Accuracy

In the treatment of disease by Reishi method stress must be laid on truth and accuracy both on the part of the agent and of the patient. Independently of the character of the patient truth must be insisted upon. The disease itself has to be examined very accurately, so as to be able to apply the Art effectively. If undue haste should lead to want of accuracy the agent discredits and injures the patient as well. Remember that the authority of TAIREIDO is at stake. With sufficient sympathy, earnestness and prudence the agent ought to persevere in being accurate. Nothing is too minute to be attended to in order to ensure accuracy. It is comparatively easy to practice this virtue with the average patient, but cases will arise where accuracy is difficult, and the agent may face a temptation to let the matter slide. In no respect should this be allowed. If once the agent permits any exception to the rule he shows himself disqualified for practicing the Art of Reishi, which above all things is the essence of Truth.

Promptitude

Accuracy without promptitude will not avail, being as ineffective as knowledge without action. The practitioner of Reishi always has a very large number of patients, and he must prepare to deal with numbers as well as with individuals. He must, therefore, learn to be deft and quick, disposing of cases without undue delay. Patients are not always patient, and if kept waiting too long will become discouraged and not return. Only experience can teach the practitioner how to get thorough his duties in the shortest possible time. But promptitude must not be at the expense of accuracy and thoroughness. The two virtues must absolutely go together with a proper frame of mind. Experience will teach the best means. Nowhere is experience as valuable as in the application of the Art of Reishi.

Boldness

It requires a brave and a bold mind to attack disease. Lack of this spirit often causes failure and so loss of life. At first, when the practitioner is without much experience in the treatment of disease, it is not so easy to command boldness of mind and attitude; yet by persistence experience will come and the day will be won. The timid and doubting practitioner will never attain results in applying the Art of Reishi. By assuming a bold and open mind and attacking the disease with courage the venturing agent will be surprised at his own success. He can thus always accomplish more than he might expect. Hesitation and wavering must not be in the category of the practitioner of the Art of Reishi. When the agent is bold and determined to Action of Reishi is induced the sooner and with greater effect, while with timidity the Action of Reishi declines. Though the Action of Reishi transcends mentality it must not be forgotten that the action may be hindered by an improper use of the mind. If one is not to hamper and restrict the Action the mind must be kept in a state of fearlessness. Water can flow over mud; but mud can be so much as to obstruct the flow of water. In the same way the Action of Reishi can be obstructed by the Action of the mind, though it is not the result of mental action but above it. The hesitating, timid mind is, therefore, fatal to proper Reishi Action. To avoid all timidity the agent, when applying the Art of Reishi, should expand his diaphragm and proceed boldly and promptly as one of the cardinal principles of effective treatment. The same virtue is essential in maintaining the other virtues already mentioned as necessary to success in the Art of Reishi. But he may possess all the other qualities and yet without boldness and firmness he will fail.

Impartiality

The principles of TAIREIDO involve observance of absolute justice and right; and, therefore, impartiality must be one of the essential virtues to success. To show preference for one patient more than another is fatal to the maintenance of a good reputation on the part of the practitioner, and indirectly affects the results of the Action of Reishi as well. Not wealth, or sex or flattery should be allowed to influence is to forfeit the confidence of the public and to lose capacity for proper application of the Art of Reishi. When the agent's centre of gravity and dignity shifts to be influenced by social position or any unworthy motive he ceases to be a successful practitioner. Men of eminence and men of humble position must be treated in exactly the same way, according to the disease to be healed. This cannot be ensured unless the agent from the beginning has his mind prepared to be above such secular influences and to observe the most scrupulous partiality in the treatment of patients. Such justice is necessary as due to the patient and also to the sacredness of Reishi. When the practitioner respects the patient and the Action of Reishi with equally profound impartiality he may hope for success.

Tenacity

It is only by tenacity that anything can be successfully accomplished. Perseverance is the condition of success. Often it happens that the last five minutes determine the issue. Therefore persist in faithfulness to the very end. It is so in war; it is so in everything. The efforts of the final moment spell victory. The diseases of the human body are enemies formidable enough; and it is only by persistence that they can be successfully attacked and driven out. This is especially so in serious chronic cases. But even slight aliments cannot be effectively cured if treated hastily or indifferently. Even in these cases it is the last few moments of treatment that count most. The agent must, therefore, be prepared to persevere in his treatment. Persistence should not be unduly prolonged, of course, but the agent should be prompt and effective. To what extent the agent should persevere must be decided by experience. Only by experience can one arrive at a correct estimate of the time and treatment necessary for the elimination of any ailment.

The twelve requisites above mentioned must be carefully observed by anyone who expects to practice the application of the Art of Reishi successfully to disease. They are preparations of the mind; and, if followed, the practitioner will be trained and well skilled in his art. At the same time it must be remembered that certain physical preparations are also essential; and these will be outlined in the succeeding chapter.

PHYSICAL PREPARATIONS NECESSARY FOR EFFECTIVE REISHI TREATMENT

As was indicated in the preceding chapter, certain physical preparations are absolutely essential to the successful practice of Reishi treatment on others. The first of these relates to the proper tension of the abdomen, the second to the clearness of the eye and the third to one's posture.

1. Tension of the Diaphragm

While acquiring the Art of Reishi no special attention need be paid to the proper way of tensing the abdomen, but when the Internal Action of Reishi is to be applied to others the proper knowledge of diaphragm action is essential. It may be speaking too strongly to assert that the proper action of the diaphragm is absolutely essential to the effectiveness of the Internal Action of Reishi when practiced on others, but such knowledge certainly adds greatly to the effectiveness of the Art of Reishi. Proper diaphragm tension is not so necessary when only a small number of patients are under treatment; but when patients are many, diaphragm tension is very important, as without it the practitioner will not be able to keep up the strength necessary to the continued operations.

Proper diaphragm tension is necessary to induction of full Reishi energy; in fact it is the source of such energy, and thereby one effects a proper application of the Reishi method. The abdomen is the seal of all spiritual power and action; and the more one has command of diaphragm action the more successful will one be in the application of the Art of Reishi. The strengthening of diaphragm action is not something that can be affected in a short time; it comes only by regular and constant practice. Any sudden attempt to gain such strength is apt to interfere with one's health. The art should be acquired gradually by systematic practice.

The best way to begin is to practice the TAIREIDO movements and processes daily. These movements are fully explained and directions given in the book on the External Action of Reishi. Among the more important of the processes there outlined is that of deep breathing. A close adherence to these Reishi formula will not only bring about full capacity for proper tension of the diaphragm but will greatly add to the general health of the Reishi practitioner. After adequate practice one finds that proper tension of the diaphragm comes naturally to the practitioner while he is engaged in the practice of the internal Action of Reishi on others for the sake of healing disease or restoring normal health or physical condition. Too much emphasis, therefore, cannot be laid on the necessity of deep breathing in acquiring mastery of diaphragm tension.

2. Clearness of the Eyes

The human eye always indicates the state of the human body. It is true of the practitioner and it is true of the patient. In applying the Internal Action of Reishi the eye should be perfectly clear. It is not good to strain the eyes overmuch, which action tends to cause fatigue of mind and body, and also tends to cause emotion or distraction of thought in the patient. With a clear eye the practitioner should try to sound the depths of truth, penetrating into the inner mysteries of the source whence he draws the power to apply the healing Art. The mouth at this time should be closed and the abdomen brought under strict tension. Clearness of vision cannot be fully attained if the mouth is open and the diaphragm is not tense. This in turn has a close relation to posture, which will be treated in the succeeding section of this chapter. For if the posture is improper the mind will not be right; and both posture and mentality have a great effect on the eyes. Without correct posture and a proper state of mind there can be no clearness of vision to penetrate the depths of Reishi Action.

3. Proper Reishi Posture

A correct posture when practicing the Internal Action of Reishi is very important; for without this a proper state of mind cannot be acquired. Though a right state of mentality is not something visible it is something of which the practitioner is conscious; but one must not suppose that a proper posture necessarily ensures a proper state of mind. One may assume a correct posture without gaining a proper state of mentality, but one cannot gain a proper state of mentality without a correct posture. By correct posture is not meant simply holding one's head erect and assuming an attitude of gravity, and so on; we mean that correct state of mentality must show itself in the whole body. For instance if the mental state causes the face or body to assume an attitude of arrogance, or aggression or any state that seems unnatural, the result will be fatal to proper application of the Art of Reishi. The posture must always be such as to reveal a correct state of mind. Correctness of posture is not something that one can expect to acquire all in a moment; one must train for it, as for anything else; and the Practice of diaphragm tension and acquiring clearness of eye will materially assist in this achievement. Without proper command of tension in the abdomen one cannot long retain correctness of posture; and if the eyes are not clear no amount of correct posturing will affect anything. One has to be careful not to make oneself ridiculous. When the abdomen is capable of great tension, and the eyes are clear and penetrating, and the posture quite correct, the whole presence assumes an attitude of majesty and power.

After the candidate for practicing the Internal Art of Reishi has mastered the above processes, and has acquired the mental and physical preparation above outlines, he is in a position to begin the successful treatment of disease. If the practitioner be indifferent or careless in regard to any of the directions and suggestions made above he will not be successful to the fullest degree. Any neglect to develop the Art of Reishi to the fullest extent is very injurious to the effectiveness of the application of the Art. Above all things the practitioner must not neglect the proper mental and physical preparation here laid down.

TREATMENT OF DISEASE BY REISHI ACTION[43]

In considering the proper method of treating disease by the application of the Internal Action[44] of Reishi it must be remembered that there are three forms of treatment: that for individuals, that for groups and that effected at a distance. Individual treatment, of course, means the application of the

[43] This chapter focuses on how Reishi, like Reiki, is used to treat disease

[44] Internal energy action inside a body versus external energy action outside

Internal Action of Reishi to separate individuals or patients. By group treatment is meant the application of the Internal Action of Reishi to a number of individuals assembled in a room, each receiving the treatment simultaneously; while distant treatment means the application of the Art to persons not in the presence of the practitioner.[45]

1. The Treatment of Individuals

There are four forms of individual treatment: pressure, massage, finger tension and palm tension[46], just as in the case of self-treatment. In the latter case the External Action of Reishi is induced by oneself and applied to oneself. But in the case under review the Action of Reishi has to be transmitted to others[47]. In these circumstances no External Action must be induced, not by finger or palm or in any other way. In the treatment of others only the Internal Action of Reishi must be induced and applied. Consequently it is very necessary that the practitioner should be well trained in the induction and practice of the Internal Action of Reishi and thus be ready and able to transmit it to others without inducing the External Action. At first it may seem to the practitioner almost impossible to know whether the External Action of Reishi is being generated and becoming active in his fingers or palms while practicing the Internal Art, but if the practitioner has fully mastered the External Action before beginning to learn the Internal Action, he will easily understand the difference. When one is master of both External Action and the Internal Action Reishi is always active within his body and proceeds from him unconsciously[48], issuing forth from him even without any intention on his part to produce it. All he has to do is to assume the proper state of mind and body[49] and apply the finger or palm in the

---

[45] These three forms are how many Reiki therapists practice nowadays

[46] In Dr Usui's 'Explanation of Usui Therapy' Hikkei he also mentions 4 forms, similar to Tanaka but with different names: Therapy of Pressing with the Hands, Stroking Therapy, Tapping Therapy, Laying on of Hands

[47] Usui also taught self-healing then healing others. Practitioners can 'impressively cure their own diseases within a short time and unerringly acquire the spiritual power to cure the diseases of others.'

[48] Usui's Hikkei says, 'The practitioner radiates a spirit and light from every part of his or her body.'

[49] Dr Usui used focus 'study the diseased part of the body for 2 or 3 minutes'

manner directed in these pages and the Internal Action will be transmitted[50]. The practitioner is absolutely forbidden to attempt to experience the Action of Reishi in his hands, as any such distraction of the mind would retard and possibly prevent the Action of Reishi. In short the practitioner must always be ready to assume a state of transcendence and allow him self to be the unconscious medium of transmitting the mysterious force that transforms and heals all disease[51].

There is no very great difference in the method adopted in treating oneself and that used in the treatment of others, the four forms above mentioned being applied in the same way in both cases. Points of divergence in treatment will be given below, as well as directions for treatment of certain ailments not already mentioned.

2. Behaviour Before and After Treatment

The Agent, always bearing strictly in mind the directions given above, usually must treat his patient while the latter is seated on a chair or lying in bed[52]. In either case the patient should be made to close the eyes, though in cases where there is mental derangement or in the treatment of children, the treatment must go on without it[53]. The practitioner should stand before the patient and then approach the latter slowly. Then he applies the finger tension method to the parts between the forehead and the elbows[54] of the patient, in intervals of two or three minutes. This treatment applies to all patients without exception. After this the pressing, massage, finger tension or palm tension methods may be applied to the parts affected, as the case demands. During the treatment the practitioner should be most careful to observe with an attitude of great solemnity and carefulness. After going through the proper treatment, the practitioner should apply the Reiyu method, as hereinafter described, after which the practitioner should assume an erect posture and announce the termination of the treatment.

---

[50] Usui's Hikkei says to breathe, massage etc, and then 'By these means inflammation will recede,' etc. The actions and results follow similar or identical patterns.

[51] Tanaka says all disease is transformed or healed. Usui in his Hikkei only says, 'A great deal of diseases displaying mental or physical conditions are cured'

[52] Nowadays there are therapy beds…

[53] Usui's Hikkei mentions 'infants and patients with serious diseases'

[54] Similar to current use of Emotional Freedom Technique (EFT)?

3. The Reiyu Method[55]

Although this method is used mostly in applying the Art of Reishi to group treatment, an explanation of it may be conveniently given here, since it is extremely useful also in treatment of individuals. To accomplish the Reiyu method the practitioner should stand erect and bring the diaphragm to firm tension, stretching the middle and fore fingers, bending the remaining fingers down as if to support the ring finger and thumb. Then the two fingers stretched out are grasped firmly by all the fingers of the left hand, and all are applied to the abdomen with firm pressure, the abdomen at the same time being under powerful tension. The tension of the abdomen must be made to coincide and unite with the tension of the fingers. The abdomen is the source of spiritual action and the fingers grasped as above are the media of the Reishi Action. When abdomen and fingers thus unite to convey the Action of Reishi the method is known as Reiyu. This method always produces most marvellous results. It has been practiced, in ignorance of its significance, by Japanese soldiers from ancient times, as part of our military art, Masters of the occult have also practiced it; but only now is its true purpose known. If the practitioner should himself be under treatment for kidney or have any affection or ailment of the abdomen he should not resort to the practice of Reiyu suddenly, but acquire mastery of it very gradually. Even to the most robust man the action of Reiyu is unadvisable until he has mastered the action of abdominal tension by deep breathing: otherwise it will affect his internal organs and brain.

4. Treatment of Special Cases

It will be seen that there is no very great difference between the methods adopted in treating oneself and in treating others by application of the Action of Reishi. Such diseases as gonorrhea, hemorrhoids and others of a very private nature, however, should be treated by the stressed finger method or by bringing the palm to tension. In cases where the palm or finger is to be applied in treatment the application must be made over the clothing and not directly on the skin. For example, when treating oneself for toothache[56] the finger under tension is pressed against the affected part, but when treating others for this ailment the stressed finger is simply held over the place and not in contact with it. The treatment should be applied for two or three minutes firmly, and then at intervals of two or three minutes, the patient keeping the mouth closed meanwhile. One should aim to apply the

---

[55] Reiyu means 'Fusion with the Spirit'

[56] Dr Usui in the Hikkei also mentions healing of toothache

method so effectively as to accomplish a cure by one treatment[57]. One should seek toothache cases as frequently as possible, as it is the best kind of case for practicing and for making advancement in the Art of healing by the Reishi method. Rheumatism[58] is likewise important for such practice and progress in the Art. This ailment can be treated by either the pressure method or by the massage method, in the same manner as for self-treatment; but sometimes the stressed finger method proves more effective. The part affected should be massaged so as to move freely in order to remove the pain gradually, though never with violence, which is bad. As in the case of toothache rheumatic pains will soon be relieved by the Reishi treatment. Chronic rheumatism, however which does not usually cause continuous pain is much more difficult to cure[59]; consequently the treatment must be very careful and persistent in order to be effective. No matter what the ailment, the practitioner has to decide for himself whether he shall apply the stressed finger or the massage method, convenience usually being the determining factor.

5. The Treatment of Mental Cases

Though one cannot usually apply mental treatment to oneself, it is quite otherwise in the case of others. There is no doubt that modern medical science has not succeeded[60] in effectively treating the affections of the mind. In fact mental cases are mostly regarded as hopeless. Yet diseases of the mind are on the increase, and it is very important to seek a proper way of relief. The removal of mental ailments is one of the most pressing necessities of life. It is not necessary, however, to give up hope, as medical science suggests[61]. The Reishi method has been found eminently successful in removing all forms of mental ailment[62]; and as the method is simple and easily secured no one should be without it that needs it.

---

[57] Usui also says cases 'have been successfully treated with just one session'

[58] Usui's Hikkei mentions healing of rheumatism too

[59] After describing how to relieve pain etc, Usui's Hikkei says, 'Chronic illnesses however, may not be dealt with in this way,' agreeing with Tanaka

[60] Usui's Hikkei agrees, saying Reiki …'has transcended modern science'

[61] Hikkei confirms Tanaka: 'Unlike psychological, hypnotherapy, and other mental treatments, Reiki does not bring with it empty implications'

[62] Hikkei lists mental ailments to be remedied, not just physical diseases

It is not so easy to treat diseases of the mind as it is to treat ordinary physical ailments. In case of mania, frenzy or convulsions[63], the eyes of the patient should be covered with a towel, which should be tied tightly over the occipital region. The arms and feet should be held down by the nurse or attendant; and then the stressed finger method should be applied to the forehead, after which the pressure method should be applied to the head, or else the massage method, including the crown of the head. Next the stomach and bowels should be treated in the same manner; and finally the back should be massaged, including the spinal cord, using the stressed finger method down the spine. The last-mentioned application should be done with vigor and energy, which usually proves more efficacious than too gentile a movement. Under such treatment the patient will become calm in a few minutes; and if not, the treatment should go on until calmness comes. When the patient does not reach a state of tranquility after due treatment, ice cold water should be applied to the soles of the feet, but no ice should be placed on the head. The disease is intensified by cold feet, and the cold application causes a reaction making the lower extremities warm, whereas if cold be applied to the head it causes a reaction toward greater heat in that region and so makes the patient worse. But this cold application should be made only to the feet of one unduly suffering from mental disease, and not to ordinary cases. But if the cold application is to be made at all it should be from the first and not after the Reishi treatment has begun. The cold application should be kept in place for at least thirty minutes and often an hour, after which the feet should be wrapped in a blanket or other warm covering[64].

Treatment of mental diseases, as above, should be applied once, twice, three or four times daily, as the case requires. Slight cases may, of course, be cured by one or two applications of the Reishi method, but for more serious cases three or four applications will be found necessary[65]. In cases of convulsion one or two applications are more efficacious than several times when the patient is calm. On this account severe mental cases are more conveniently treated in the hospital. If the state of the patient be calm it is unnecessary to cover the eyes with a towel. Ordinary cases can be healed by the above in one or two weeks, though no period can be definitely named, since cases differ so widely. There are cases of hysteria, especially in women, which are as difficult to cure as the usual mental diseases; and for

---

[63] Also mentioned in Usui's Hikkei

[64] Tanaka has unusually in-depth detail on how to help specific conditions. Usui and modern therapists rarely detail how to help one specific condition

[65] Hikkei agrees saying chronic conditions usually require several sessions

such patients the same treatment must be applied. In fact all cases of mental derangement can be treated much the same. For melancholia the same treatment is given, except that the eyes need not be covered nor the limbs held down. In case of mental derangement the patient should be made always to practice deep breathing, which always much assist the treatment, causing, as it does, decrease of the diaphragm power in the patient. Mental cases may be judged by the ability to count. If a mental case has any idea of number the ailment is improving. To be able to count up to six shows good progress in recovery. If the patient can count up to ten his case is not difficult to cure[66].

In this way all diseases of the mind can be treated and successfully cured. There are more ailments of the mind than are generally recognised as such. Nearly all eccentricity or abnormal enthusiasm shows some derangement of the mind. People who become too zealous or excited over religion, politics, art or science usually need treatment by Reishi; and frequently a patient can be prevented from going into a state of madness by proper Reishi treatment in time. In an age of keen competition and undue excitement like the present it is most desirable that everybody should have the benefit of Reishi treatment in order to keep the mind well balanced to endure the stress of daily life[67]. To be able to apply the Action of Reishi to the self or to receive such treatment from others able to administer it, is a great preventative to the ills of mental and physical existence.

6. Treatment of Groups

By treatment of groups is meant the treatment of several individuals in a room at one time. There need be no limit to the number of persons so treated, nor is it necessary that they should all have the same ailment. The application of the power that regulates and ress the human system, no matter what is the cause of its irregularity or incapacity; and so it is possible to apply the Art to any number of persons at the same time, even though each may have different ailment. Such treatment must, of course, be given by a practitioner who is well skilled in the Art of Reishi. The success of the treatment will depend largely on how fully the practitioner has developed the Reiyu method, which requires a well developed diaphragm.

In treating a group the patients are made to stand in the proper posture and to close their eyes. Then they are treated by Reiyu method for about half an hour. When the Action of Reishi is transmitted to the individuals they will

---

[66] Again Tanaka gives rare insight to adjust treatment for specific conditions

[67] Nowadays research evidence shows Reiki can balance and relieve stress

experience a very pleasant feeling. In any of them had pain or soreness, it will have gone. During the process the agent must preserve a most solemn and sacred attitude, else the Action will not be equally effective on all the members of the group. Usually the Action of Reishi will be fully experienced some ten or twenty minutes after the commencement of the operation; so that the first fifteen minutes the agent must be particularly prudent and careful in regard to formulae. Some patients find great difficulty in controlling themselves during the operation; but the agent must warn them before beginning of treatment not to open their eyes no matter how much they want to do so, and to keep, by all means, the proper posture assigned to them until the end of the operation. It is better, therefore, never to include children or adults in great pain in group treatment by Reishi method. Those suffering from mental trouble had also better be excluded. Anything that disturbs the members of the group is likely to defeat the efforts of the practitioner to accomplish a cure. The agent must keep himself in proper condition for effective work, commanding an attitude of absolute stability and complete self-transcendence.

Individual treatment can be undertaken immediately after group treatment and *vice versa,* though the practitioner must bear in mind that he cannot expect successful results unless he is in proper condition, especially as to training and full development in the Art of Reishi[68].

7. Combination Group Treatment

Sometimes treatment is more successful having the members of the group stand in circle with the practitioner in the middle. The members face the agent, standing apart from one another and holding each others' hands. The agent then practices the Reiyu method for about thirty minutes, during which he moves around the line of figures before him from one to three times, very slowly. Another way is to begin the practice of Reiyu by moving forward to within an inch or so of the circles, then having the circle move around the agent toward the right. In this operation most of the patients will soon be relieved of whatever trouble they were suffering from. Of course no very serious cases of mental derangement, or great pain, or children, can be treated in this way. Patients seriously affected with tuberculosis also should not be treated after this manner; nor indeed should any case of contagious

[68] This method of group treatment is rarely used, maybe because, as Tanaka states, successful results are not achieved unless therapist is trained fully

disease be taken into the circle. Even those with a cough had better be excluded[69].

It is also sometimes a good plan for the practitioner to join in the circle as a member, taking the hands of those on either side of him, by which he can transmit the Internal Action of Reishi to the other members of the circle[70]. This method is particularly open to an agent who has advanced to the fourth degree in the practice of the Art of Reishi.

8. Treatment at a Distance

Those who have not advanced to the fourth degree[71] in the practice of the Art of Reishi should not attempt the application of the Art at a distance.[72] Of course Reishi, not unlike electricity, transcends the laws of space and time[73], and it produces a spiritual action in the patient simultaneously with the beginning of the Action of Reishi in the agent for purpose of treatment, though such action is not visible[74]. Some patients show the influence of the External Action of Reishi greatly after treatment, but the proportion of these is rather small[75]. Nor do the patients under treatment experience any particular sensation[76]. Their illness simply vanishes before the Reishi treatment without their being otherwise conscious of any change[77]. If recovery is gradual they will experience improvement after every treatment[78]. Whether the patient is aware of being treated at a distance or not benefit will be experienced after the agent has performed the Reishi treatment.

---

[69] As with some current Reiki Masters such as Allan Sweeney, Tanaka lists conditions that are not appropriate for therapy

[70] This is similarly practiced now, including by Hiroshi Doi as Reiki Mawashi. Perhaps there is a lineage for Mawashi going back to Dr Usui?

[71] Takata had 3 degrees, as do most masters. Tanaka had 4 degrees, Usui 7

[72] A system of knowledge, with distant healing only taught after basics. Usui also taught distant healing

[73] Masters now teach how hon sha ze sho nen can heal thru time and space

[74] For current scientific evidence see Dr Daniel Benor's 'Healing Research'

[75] Shows Tanaka is honest about failure rates

[76] Unlike hands-on therapy, distant patients do not feel the energy

[77] Students in my class practice cure family at home who hadn't realized

[78] Like Usui, Tanaka had many patients to help him assess how they react

For distant treatment the agent should be in possession of the patient's photograph[79] or handwriting, which though not absolutely necessary[80], is rather convenient as an objective or reminder. Any photograph will do, whether recent or not, either in group or single, bust or full length. The patient should be required to make a formal application to the agent, with his name, address, age and ailment as well as the actual state of progress of the disease[81]. When the time for treatment comes the agent simply stands up and places the photograph or the handwriting on a table. Then he reads the application, specially noting what is said of the ailment to be a treated[82]. When he feels he has mastered the statement he begins the practice of Reiyu for about five minutes at most[83]. To him these five minutes will seem an age, and he will find it difficult to keep on, but he must persist[84]. But the method must not induce stopping the breath too long, as this is able to injure the brain and kidneys[85]. During Reiyu practice the agent should breathe at least twice in a minute. The strain thus renders it necessary that the agent should cultivate perfection in the art of assuming an attitude of complete self-transcendence, without which successful treatment is not possible[86]. The giving of treatment at a distance is excellent practice in acquiring the art of self-transcendence, as the agent is not influenced by the patient's presence in any way, and so is free to develop his natural capacity uninterrupted.

When the agent assumes an attitude of self-transcendence and begins to practice the Reiyu method his treatment of the distant patient will at once begin to take effect. The form to be gone through for effective treatment is the same in all cases, though the agent must have a different record before

---

[79] Photographs are often used by distant healers nowadays

[80] Reiki masters still teach distant healing with or without photographs

[81] Tanaka used records for research evidence of improvement

[82] Focus was on patient and need. Some now think of anything…

[83] Not too different to now. Many masters say 10 minutes at most

[84] Again, focus was key to success

[85] Not used nowadays. Maybe it was found to be too dangerous

[86] Edgar Cayce, 1930s, said healing in semi-trance overcame his era's low vibrations. Today's higher vibrations mean trance is not needed

him for each case to be treated[87]. The agent must send previous notice of time or treatment to the patient, when possible, though the necessary elimination of this is requirement does not interfere with the efficacy of the treatment. The patient should be requested to report his condition to the agent every four days, but the absence of such report need not interfere with the treatment.

9. Notice of Improvement before Treatment

Sometimes it happens that the patient sends notice of improvement experienced before the agent has actually gone through the operation for treatment at a distance. This often causes the agent much perplexing thought. There are two ways of interpreting this. One is to conclude that the patient, having applied for treatment, is naturally expecting some change, and his mentality is so influenced that the Action of Reishi is induced, causing his trouble to improve[88]. Another way of looking at it is to assume that the agent has unconsciously transmitted the Internal Action of Reishi after hearing of the case, for Reishi transcends time and space[89] in its effect on others and its influence will coincide with the mental or spiritual state of the patient, producing the improvement experienced. This effect of Reishi is something seen in cases of mental ailment or children's' ailments for which application has been made for treatment. The improvement they experience prior to treatment is due to the effect of the Action of Reishi unconsciously transmitted by the agent to whom application for treatment was made. Most of the cases that apply for treatment are, of course, serious cases that cannot reach the agent; and when such cases experience improvement, they naturally can see no connection with the agent, or with Reishi, but the improvement is due to Reishi nevertheless[90].

WE believe in the existence
of *Tairei*, which we not only
understand by means of
intellect but feels also as it
really is TEIREIDO

---

[87] Tanaka kept clinical records, as did Hayashi, and many current therapists. It is unlikely that Dr Usui (who comes between Tanaka and Hayashi and was also interested in outcomes) would not also have kept clinical records

[88] This is currently called a placebo response

[89] This statement coincides with current science that all is in the present

[90] Research since 1970s shows such health effects of distant healing

TAIREI

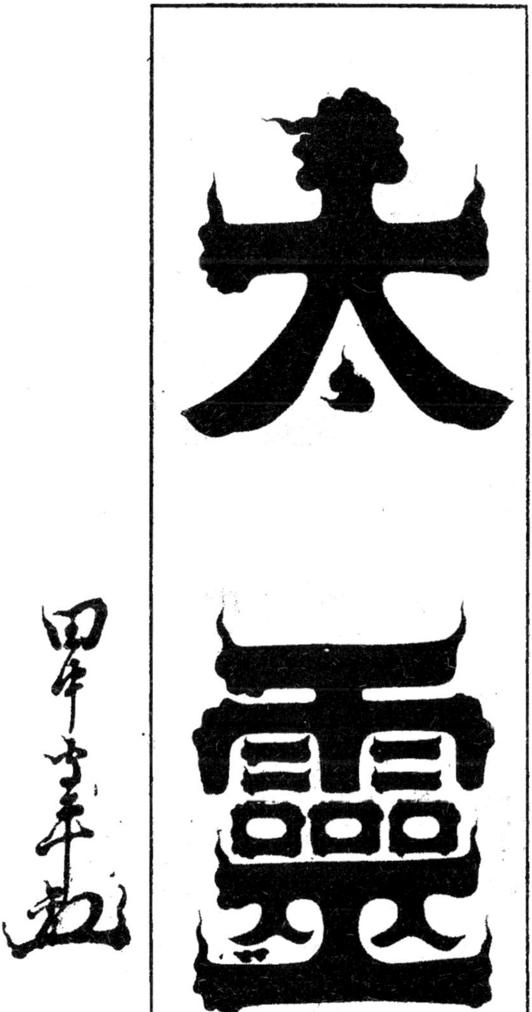

Hand Writing of The Founder

Part I

A NEW REVELATION

The Revelation

By TAIREIDO, or the Great Spirit, is revealed to those able to perceive it a Divine Light and Power, gleaming through the utmost limits of earth and heaven, guiding the world and enveloping the universe. The Light[91] and Power of TAIREI are eternal and omnipresent, the primal source of existence from which the world draws all sustenance.

Man's inability to perceive this Light and receive this Power leaves the human world still dark and weak even after ages of existence. Men are everywhere helplessly adrift like things of chance on the whirlpool of time and know no rest or hope. Driven hither and thither these human atoms are lost to the way of life and safety. TAIREI holds up the light and throws out the life-line to rescue from the drifting and the dark all who believe.

O people of the earth, will you not heed the call and come where you can be prepared to discern this Light and receive this Power, wherein is your ark of safety? Will you not abandon the seven-fold falsehoods of the mind and the three-fold vices of the flesh, and look upon this Light that it may transfuse you, giving you the saving Power in which you may abide forever? Then alone will the path of Truth and Life and Peace be yours! Then and by this alone will life be whole and perfect. In TAIREI only is to be found solution for the ills of time!

WE believe in the nature of *Tairei* which consists in being free from limitations of time and space, existence and non-existence.

[91] Usui may be referring to the same light in the 'hikkei.'

The Creed

I believe in TAIREI, the GREAT SPIRIT, the source of all things in heaven and earth; and to the principles and precepts of TAIREI I affirm my utmost loyalty and obedience. I venerate the Sovereign, value the State, honour my parents and ancestors, manage well my family affairs, love mankind, strive to uplift society, respect all living creatures, foster the life of the universe, recognise its absoluteness, emulate its discrimination, believe firmly and carefully in truth, reject thoughtless doubt, observe impartiality and justice, apprehend and comprehend in my body the potentialities of the universe, labor for excellence, act generously, behave discreetly in speaking, writing and in deportment, being polite, courteous and cordial to all men. I even maintain a magnanimous attitude, cherish faith, obey order, and observe frugality of life and assiduity in business, doing nothing without due discretion, thinking deeply and keeping firm to resolution. I cultivate grace of character and perfection of personality, encouraging vigor of body and discipline of spirit, acting in harmony with character and promoting development of intellect. In essentials I am always inflexible and in temper indomitable, having the pride that goes with proper self-respect. Abandoning the seven falsehoods of the mind and the three vices of the flesh I return to my true self and reveal in my body the divinity that produced me and shapes my ends. I perceive the chances of life and deal prudently with its accidents. I follow systematically the path of progress, knowing when to move and when to stop, indifferent to praise or blame. I go through with what is undertaken, aiming chiefly at the establishment of truth and attainment of perfection.

Fundamental Doctrines of TAIREI

I As to TAIREI:

1. Man must apprehend and believe in TAIREI, the Ultimate Reality.
2. TAIREI is free from limitations of space and time, existence and non-existence, transcending all things.
3. TAIREI comprises perfect unity between the thinking subject and the object thought of, and is the final cause of all powers of numbers or nullity.
4. TAIREI is the sum and substance of all truth and goodness, comprising all perfection.
5. TAIREI is the true Deity.

II As to the Universe:

1. The universe is product of one all-pervading principle called REISHI, which is an emanation of TAIREI and the means by which the latter manifests itself in creation.

2. REISHI manifests itself in action, the form of which is symbolized by the sign 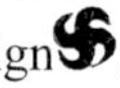; the alternation of all transient phenomena in the world is the action of REISHI and perfectly done.

3. All things come into being of necessity through the categorical imperative of TAIREI.

4. All things thus brought into being are rational, proceeding, as they do, from the Divine Will of TAIREI, and they have a divine significance.

5. Universal phenomena move, revolve around and return to TAIREI existing beyond time and space; thence they issue and thence they return, repeating the same process through infinity.

III As to Society:

1. Society is the absolute form resulting from character and capacity of the universe in motion, a manifestation of the Divine Spirit.

2. Of the various communal forms mankind is the highest and ultimate.

3. The Power and capacity to form into communities or societies is inherent in the individuals composing such aggregations, the power for organizing underlying the nature of the community as a whole.

4. The social nature of the community is real and perfect, and independent of all determinations of space and time.

5. The will and functions of a community move according to rhythmic spiritual laws.

IV As to the State:

1. The State is the most perfect form in which the social nature of the community manifests itself.

2. The State is the only organized form by which the order and discipline necessary to human society can be maintained.

3. The paramount purpose of the State is to establish and maintain order among its members.

4. The authority which the State exercises over its members must be absolute.

5. There should be but one State, and the various states now existing should be unified toward this end.

V As to the Individual:

1. The life of each individual is a gift from TAIREI.

2. Every individual is an organized form completely manifesting the nature and power of TAIREI.

3. All individuals, the living and the dead form one complete system or whole.

4. The individual must find his natural condition of existence in family life; the relation of man and wife is the starting point or base of social existence, the couple forming the unit of society and the manifestation of its character and capacity.

5. Of all created things the individual is the highest and the head.

WE believe that *Tairei* is wholly true and good.

Some Precepts of TAIREI

1. Have unwavering faith in TAIREI and venerate profoundly the Source of all things. One should become increasingly conscious of one's transcendence above the visible world. Assume a temper of absoluteness to things and be able to stand where discrimination is possible. Reveal in life the whole truth. Live the divinity that is in you!

2. Not only manifest the divine character within your body but develop thereby a greater capacity for divinity. Obey carefully the law by which divine character is retained and revealed, the capacity being symbolized in the sign, which means perfection. Fail not to observe the laws and precepts of TAIREI. Cultivate rigidly a true insight into the significance of things and

be able to apprehend the divine will of Tairei. Note the affinity of all moving phenomena and the reason of it: how there is movement, revolution and return to the source, forgetting not the good effect thereof.

3. Be social; and let society be the sphere of manifesting your character. Understand thoroughly the general character and capacity of society, and act in consonance therewith, being especially careful to note the divine aspect of social life.

4. Let your highest character be manifested in national life, ever rendering some effective service to your country. Observe and faithfully follow the ultimate purposes of the nation. Obey the highest authority of the nation. Labor to promote the unity of all nations in one great State.

5. Preserve carefully your health and your life. Let your real self return to great All-self and have real communion with TAIREI. Honour your ancestors and your parents and foster your children. Manage discretely your household and let husbands and wives live in peace and harmony. Above all things cherish the Spirit of the Universe, in which you live and move and have your being!

WE believe that a community
is the matter-of-fact form of
existence of things that partake
of the power of the Almighty.

Intellectual Apprehension of TAIREIDO

1. General Considerations

Man is self-conscious being. He looks up into the illimitable sky and beholds the innumerable stars in their brightness: he feels lost in the presence of such immensity. He then casts his eyes down to the vast earth and sees it swarming with helpless moving creatures as innumerable as the stars, of which he is but one. He cannot avoid some inference as to the significance of his own existence thus thrown between the boundless expanse of earth and heaven. Has human life any value? If so, has it more value than other forms of life? What is Man's origin? What his destiny? Whither does he desire to go?[92] Transiency is the mark of all things: change is to be expected. Through immemorial ages the heavens and the earth have undergone numerous transformations. Yet the earth still exists and man persists upon its surface. Amid all the mutations of time man is haunted by questions as to the significance of his life and its final end. But has any human mind ever succeeded in evolving a solution of life's enigma from its own self-consciousness? Buddha said: "Throughout the heavens and the earth I alone am holy;" and Jesus Christ, claiming to be the Son of God, said: "I am the Way, the Truth and the Life: no man cometh to the Father but by me!" These two sages represent the sum total of human consciousness as to Man's place in the universe. Yet they do not quite seem to coincide as to TAIREI: the ABSOLUTE TRUTH, from all the limitations of human individuality. Is the question of questions in regard to human life then insoluble? Hitherto it has been thought so. But we shall see!

2. The Supreme Question

Though the vast majority of the world's population is too busy struggling for mere existence to pause for such a question as that relating to the significance of existence, the whole tendency of the age is urging a prompt solution of the problem. When man reflects calmly on the number of his days and seeks to know his end, he cannot but feel anxious and sad and ponder on some way toward relief. That man should exist only for toil to get food and raiment, and be moved only by his passions, from birth to death, seems intolerable to contemplate. Is this the whole truth of human life? If the struggle of life is for mere existence how can any value be attached to it? If life be no more than toil and passion what does it amount to? No: life is something more than a matter of food and clothing and passion: it is a

[92] These are classic questions asked by most serious Reiki practitioners

fundamental problem down deep in the life of every individual in the universe, back of all his breathing; of the aggregate of individuals in society, on the surface of all their breathing; and of the source and essence of life, both on the surface and behind the veil.

3. Human Life

Man is born he knows not why; nor does he know the true reason of his death. Yet he is born and dies nevertheless. What then are the real causes of birth and death? It is an ancient adage that man knows little of life and less of death. Yet there is nothing that he has a greater desire to know! Not only so, but man has an unceasing desire to transcend both life and death. The paramount question then is how to know the why and the wherefore of life and death and how to Transcend them. To what degree, if any, is such transcension possible? To say that we know life and death and still say we cannot transcend them is to say we do not know them. And even if we succeed in transcending the realities of life and death and yet do not do so to the utmost degree possible, it cannot be truly said that we have solved the all-important question of what human life is.

4. Origin and Destiny

The long unceasing procession of life and death seems a great mystery. A hundred years ago we were not; a hundred years hence and we are no more. Thus the human form, with all its marvellous organisation, comes and goes; and what of it? Man's life at the longest is but brief. How did man come to have the form given him, and what is its real destiny? Whence comes this life of ours that seldom survives a hundred years?

Whither is it speeding? To many the origin of life is one's parents and its destiny is the tomb. But whence did the parents obtain life? Life came from parents again; and so one might go back to the primal origin of man. This is a matter for profound and useful study. Equally important is the study of life's destiny. The destiny of life must be something higher than the tomb. It rests with each individual whether he will make his life of temporal or eternal value; whether out of his mortal body he shall evolve an immortal life. Man therefore should study carefully his origin and destiny.

5. Mutations and Survival

The universe is in a state of unceasing transition. Amid the flux and flow of things man too is changing. Even while the mind thinks about it the change is going on, even in the mind itself. The present becomes the past before we have time to think about it. Thus while we are occupied in explaining a condition, it is past and exists no more. We are left talking about what does not exist. The past, the present and the future are never quite the same. The transiency of creation is its normal condition. Man too is involved in the endless process: he cannot stand aloof. He is always coming and going, moving along the path of life and death in endless transition.

6. Primal Substance

What is the cause of the phenomena of eternal transition and change? It is the primal substance that pervades all things. There can be no phenomenon apart from substance; and substance cannot be observed apart from phenomena. Man must, therefore, recognise this Great Substance that is the cause of all phenomena, including man himself. This Substance is the cause of all change in the Universe. To this cause also we owe all the phenomena of the natural world. This Substance, or Being, is infinite in space and time, supreme above all existence. It neither increases nor decreases amid the universal transitoriness, but remains above and beyond all mutation.

7. TAIREI

When the human mind contemplates profoundly the origin of change: of creation and decay, of life and death, the appearance and disappearance of individual beings on earth, it inevitably becomes convinced of the reality of the Great Substance, or Being, that is the cause of it all; and man becomes conscious that he is the product of that same illimitable Power and Life, possessing alike its unlimited power and duration. He realizes having a Substance that was never born and will never die. By such a process of thought man can perceive the origin and cause of life and death, and can place himself beyond them.

This Great Substance, or Being, is in these pages called TAIREI, representing in all completeness the attributes of perfection. The whole universe was formed and society brought into existence for the revelation of the Truth of TAIREI, which is always and everywhere supreme. All the comings and goings of transition and transmutation are the action of this Substance, which transcends the limits of space and time. All phenomena are impressed with the perfect Truth of TAIREI: its image is seen upon creation. This Substance binds together the present and the past and the future: there is no disintegration. In the social side of universal life is the impress of TAIREI most clearly and actively seen. Man is of this Substance, possessing its character and capacity, and may rely confidently on the reality of his relations therewith.

TAIREI is related to us in the same way that we are to one another. We come from the same source whence all things issue; and thus like the rest of creation man is cast between the heaven the earth, undergoing the changes of birth and death, of arrival and return. Man is related to TAIREI as really and truly as TAIREI is to the universe. The Great Substance is ever inbreathed by us and by all the communal life of man. It is the life of the physical body and the social body, the family and the state. Life comes into contact and communion with TAIREI through breathing.

8. Universality

Humanity is an essential part of the universe issuing forth from TAIREI, the Supreme Substance of things; and by contact with TAIREI man commands the transcendent character of his origin. Man is more than one individual: he partakes of universal being. He is an individual as a member of society; a being of universal character in relation to the universal and a social character man reveals the true nature of the character of TAIREI. When man is trained to perceive this truth there is nothing to prevent his possessing all that is of true worth in heaven and earth, for then he has the Power of TAIREI. Then man is TAIREI and TAIREI is man. The Truth of TAIREI is then ours; and our words and deeds are the doing of TAIREI. Man is the universe and the universe is man. Society is the individual and the individual is society. TAIREI is the measure of all things; and in TAIREI man is likewise. The universe revolves and evolves through endless change, just as man does, and so does society, and both are the efforts of universal life. What man then proposes is the purpose of TAIREI, and the proposals and purpose of the latter are those of man. The object or purpose of the universe is Man's too; and Man's aims are those of the universe. The ideal of society will then be the ideal of the individual, and the ideal of the individual that of society. Man's ideals will become significant only as they are in harmony with the purpose of the universe; and human activity has value only as it fulfils the good of society. Thus the true end of life can be known only by submission to TAIREI.

9. Eternal Life

What is the supreme purpose of the Great Spirit, TAIREI? What is the true ideal of society, the true object of the universe? Progress is the aim of the universe, equality and harmony from the ideal of society, and perfection and truth are purposes of TAIREI for all things. In every created thing there is some evidence of progress: in the tiniest petal of a flower, even in a drop of water. If this be true of the lower forms of creation it is much truer of man. The strife after more equality and harmony can be seen even among birds and beasts. Much more is it true of men. Every tree and stone has its lesson for those willing to learn. This must be much truer of men! Progress should be leading feature of social life, and by harmonious growth perfection should be promoted. The real purpose of life, therefore, is perfection and truth: to make mankind truly one with the rest of the universe: to make society one with TAIREI which it seeks to live and express. Man is destined to reveal in himself the divine character and capacity, the divine perfection and truth that are given by TAIREI. Man has to believe firmly in the possibility of such attainment, and then seek it. When the divine and vital bond that binds the whole universe together is truly functioning in human society the end purpose of existence will have been achieved. But man has to learn how to get rid of that individualism that prevents his union with the universal character, so that humanity may be one with the perfection and supremacy of TRUTH. When man attains unto the absolute Truth of TAIREI, when the Truth of the universe becomes the Truth of society, then character will be perfect, independent of the limits of space and time. Man then will emit that divine light of the existence of which he is yet but dimly conscious. He will possess and use the Light and Power of TAIREI.

Part II

Science of Reishi

1. Significance of the System

TAIREIDO aims to correct the physical, mental and spiritual inaccuracies of man so as to produce perfection of character and condition which alone is consistent with truth and happiness. The destiny of man on this earth is to be brought completely into harmony with the way of the Great Spirit of all things.[93] People are constantly under the influence and consequently the evil of mistaken ideas because they lack the system of reason and action which the Science of Reishi imparts. When man learns the Way of the Great Spirit and practices that Way his whole being will be in harmony with TAIREI, and he will enjoy the happiness of perfect existence.

To this desirable end every human being may come by subjecting to the process of Reishi, the active power of TAIREI. Through Reishi which is the means of operation, the individual is enabled to realize his thought by putting it perfectly into practice. Thought and theory are of no value until they can be practically applied to actual human life. Essential thought belongs to man, and he alone can attain unto its consummation. By the

---

[93] Sounds similar to Usui-sensei's description of his Reiki Therapy.

process of Reishi the ideals of TAIREI may be known and practically applied, the individual actually acquiring the power of TAIREI. By the process of Reishi true ideas are materialised, so to speak; and only as the individual can this live his ideas is he perfect man.

The process of Reishi, therefore, makes the ideas of TAIREI possible of realization in every Man's existence. Reishi teaches man how to cultivate the divine ideas of TAIREI and how to develop his reasoning power so as to put these ideas into practical application. It is paramount, therefore, that the individual man shall acquire true knowledge of the process of Reishi that he may have the power to think and live a true life and lead his fellow men along the same path of light. It is then that man comes to a practical realization of the divinity that is his birthright: man is divinised, as it were, because the science of TAIREIDO is his and the process of Reishi the active principle of his existence. By this knowledge and this power every man can be sane and whole in all his parts, living a true life.

2. The Process of Reishi

Reishi is the active principle of TAIREI, the Great Spirit.[94] It is the process by which the Divine life and power work. By Reishi man acquires the knowledge of TAIREI and how to apply it to the daily needs of life. Human history is full of attempts at gaining such knowledge and power, most of these attempts toilsome and disappointing, covering long years of mental and physical struggle with unwearied application and no satisfaction or efficacy in the end. Such efforts of man after his divine birthright usually demand great spiritual faith and great physical endeavor, showing Man's belief in great possibilities yet unattained. Reishi, the true process of realization, however, demands no creed save reason and the action of reason. Like the science of electricity, once the knowledge is acquired the rest is easy: it works itself once given the means.

Reishi is the source of all life: in it the fusing of the spiritual and material becomes real. It is open to the rich and the poor, and by it the prince and the pauper alike must live.

Though the process of Reishi has but recently come to be accurately known and applied, its action has been experienced among men for ages. Reishi is potentially in all created things. Knowledge of Reishi is how to use a power within you, of which TAIREI is the origin. If it were within the province of

[94] Similar to an explanation of Reiki taken from Takata-sensei's diary: 'a universal force from the Great Divine Spirit'

man to apply the force within a grain of radium he could do marvellous things: he can do still greater things once he commands the knowledge of the power within himself. It is this that the founder of the system of TAIREIDO has discovered and now desires to share with his fellow men. The method is simple and exact: any one can acquire it. The results are so convincing that no one who has become acquainted with them has ever hesitated to go on and become a follower of TAIREIDO. The most stubborn sceptic must recognise truth when he sees it, and the results of the operation of Reishi are truth, living truth.

But even the greatest power is powerless until the means of its application are acquired and put into practice. TAIREIDO does not reveal the Reishi without means, and more than electricity or any other power does. The science of Reishi affords a simple and easy process by which the power is brought under Man's command and use. All ignorant of this process will be as void of the power as if it did not exist, except incidentally; for all power is from TAIREI; but only those acquainted with the science of Reishi have it at rational and conscious command.

3. Reishi Different from Mind-Healing and Faith-cure

The process of Reishi is quite different from the many methods adopted by various cults in modern times, such as mind-healers, faith-cure and those who work by hypnotism[95]. These have their origin in the possibilities which TAIREIDO offers in the human body as a basis for its true operation, but they in no way compare with the science of Reishi as the power by which TAIREI truly works for Man's good. The means resorted to by these cults are purely mental, and the science of Reishi does not admit the possibility of producing spiritual phenomena by mental action. It is not denied that certain types of illness or bodily affection may be relieved or cured by mental suggestion or action; but if the cure be real, we hold that it is due to the action of Reishi outside of any mental action. The action of Reishi is often applied unconsciously, the practitioner meanwhile thinking that the result is due to his own mind. In the same way we live and move and have our being in Reishi daily without any effort of mind. In hypnotic processes and practice of mesmerism the good results are due to Reishi and not to mental action. The relation between Reishi and such mental processes is purely accidental and not essential. In the same way human ailments are sometimes cured or relieved by religious faith. Here we come to something nearer to

---

[95] Usui's Hikkei uses almost identical words - Reiki is not the same as faith healing, other methods of healing, (kiaijutsu can be termed mind-healing), or hypnotism.

the action of Reishi: for there is no doubt that ardent faith does excite the action of Reishi. But in all cases of real cure the result is due to the action of Reishi and not to any mental action[96].

Similar phenomena appear in relation to material treatment of disease. In pathology it is readily admitted that the action of medicine is helped by the faith of the patient. If there is belief in the efficacy of the treatment the results are usually more hopeful. Distrust, on the contrary, diminishes the prospects of improvement. Sometimes pabulums of practically no medical value have been known to affect beneficially patients who had much faith in them. We hold that such results are due to Reishi rather than to the mental action of the patient. It is Reishi which accomplishes the good results of all treatment of disease, whether mental, spiritual or material. This is why the action of proper medicine is the same whether the patient trusts or distrusts the remedy. Medicine therefore sometimes may excite or enliven the faculty through which Reishi works and a cure may be accomplished; but conscious exercise of that faculty is the normal and effective course offered by TAIREIDO.

Reishi is always the cause of the beneficial change or cure no matter what the treatment, though practitioners may erroneously attribute the good results to their mental, spiritual or material action. Those ignorant of the nature of Reishi often argue as to the comparative merits of mental, spiritual or material treatment, not knowing that none of these treatments necessarily conflict. All that any treatment can hope to do is to give Reishi a chance to work. The best and surest means of accomplishing this is by following the science of Reishi. All treatments, so far as they appear to be successful, are partial applications of Reishi. All treatments, however, are uncertain and imperfect compared with TAIREIDO and the science of Reishi, which apply the action of Reishi directly and efficaciously.

In the application of Reishi, however, mental or material processes are not resorted to, the faculty of cure being excited by the direct application of Reishi. Reishi cures as nature cures, for Reishi is nature. The action of Reishi is independent of both mind and matter. The tendency of the present age is toward the super-mental and the super-material, and Reishi is in harmony with that tendency. It is a trend toward the Almighty. Reishi is the origin of both mind and matter; and this is why the science of Reishi is paramount in human life.

---

[96] Mental action creates Reishi, so it's Reishi that cures, not mental action

The science of Reishi is not for the treatment of disease alone: it is for all life, and the essential principal of true existence. Understanding the process of Reishi one can realize the most mysterious phenomena and appreciate the most baffling facts in experience. Indeed none of the processes of life are successful without the action of Reishi. It is the active principal and motive power of all true life processes whether artificial or natural; and therefore the application of this science to life surpasses all other treatment or resource or method. It is applied to disease that is one of the greatest obstructing features in human life, and man will give anything to get rid of disease. This is why Reishi has become especially famous in the treatment of disease; but as the essential principle of life Reishi is as necessary to the well as to the sick. If a man feels no need of anything he at least must prepare to deal with disease when it comes, either to him self or others. For the sake of his fellow men, if not for his own, he is bound to know the way of Reishi. There is no man that does not want all the perfection and advantage that life can afford; and as Reishi offers the best within the reach of man, every man must desire to become acquainted with it.

Part III

Action of Reishi

As already suggested, the action of Reishi comprises the fundamental processes of life, transcending all human mentality and physiology: which are the result of Reishi. Every living thing exists, thrives and fulfils its rightful functions by means of Reishi, and no phenomena of life are possible without it. Within all mental and physical phenomena proceeds the action of Reishi, which is the fundamental basis of all life functions. What man now must understand is that this power always working within may also be made to work without, provided one knows the proper means. It is very important that the attention be now given to this twofold action of Reishi.

1. External Action of Reishi

When the external action of Reishi is spoken of we mean action on the surface. By this action the body and limbs move automatically and naturally yet in a manner quite different from the ordinary phenomena of life, transcending the laws of mentality and physics. In the history of human development it has been found that human beings by severe bodily discipline have been able to do wonderful things physically, but few have been able thus to command the powers of the body freely and naturally.

Even those approaching such attainments have been quite unconscious of the fundamental action of life, regarding it as a mysterious phenomenon due to divine interposition. They have never been able to realize that such power is spontaneous and not the result of outside interference. They have been content to thank God for the manifestations of His power and go on to stronger faith in religion.

In sense such an experience is a manifestation of divine power. That is only a reasonable view when man believes he has been touch by the Absolute. The idea of God, however, has been hitherto a very vague one, the main notion being that of personification, so that men may conceive of God as possessing men. But this is quite different from the true idea of God. Man can easily recognise the fact that a personal God takes possession of him. But what man most needs to understand is the fundamental action of life: that is, the external action of Reishi, which is quite independent of man being taken possession of by a personal God. As Reishi is the natural process of life man may command it without reference to God, because no life, not even man himself can exist without its presence. To speak of being thus independent of the favour of God may seem strange to ears accustomed to religious phraseology, but when one realizes that men without religion have in them the fundamental bases of life just the same as those religiously devoted to God, the truth of the contention will be apparent.

The actions of Reishi are the sum-total of the force of TAIREI acting in accordance with the laws of perfect truth and transcending all things. In the broadest sense of the term TAIREI may be understood as God, and the science of Reishi the divine science. But the action of Reishi proceeding from its source in TAIREI must be presented through the human body, the chief medium of its manifestation. Reishi is simply the TAIREI, or Great Spirit, manifesting itself. The presence of Reishi may indeed sometimes be experience by accident; but its true realization and utilization depends on knowledge of the fundamental means by which Reishi works.

Such incidental experiences of the external action of Reishi as have been known in human history in the past have been known to occur for the most part during periods of fasting. Such experiences have been mine too during times of rigid spiritual culture, once especially in the woods at Gifu. It is a well known experience that fasting and certain spiritual action are inseparable. It is not that the action of Reishi is due to fasting, but during physical abstinence one can perceive the action of Reishi more clearly. The reason is that through the habit of centuries the body's dependence on food has become hereditary; and when this sustenance is removed for any appreciable time, the body calls in another force to sustain it, namely,

Reishi. This shows that something other than food sustains life and that Reishi is the primal source of existence. While man partakes of food regularly the action of Reishi is internal and he is unconscious of its action; but when he goes without food long enough to require assistance, the action of Reishi becomes external and he becomes conscious of it. This is why fasting is very important in treatment of illness, as all physicians acknowledge; for fasting gives Reishi a better chance to operate in setting to work the restorative faculties. Even in such treatment, however, the action of Reishi is for the most part internal rather than external. When the action is wholly external the result is more prompt and complete.

Since it is true that fasting and the action of Reishi have a close relation it is not to be wondered at that religious devotees have from time immemorial practiced the habit as a necessary form of devotion; but after all it is only an unwitting testimony to an unconscious effort after knowledge of Reishi, or the action of God on human life. Not unnaturally, therefore, in teaching the fundamental principles of Reishi we prescribe fasting from one to two weeks at a time, according to physical capacity[97]. But it is quite possible to acquire the science of Reishi without fasting, if one faithfully follows directions. Even in fasting there must be some order and method; for one does not experience the process of Reishi simply by abstaining from food. Hitherto men merely fasted, and thereby often injured their health, but now they follow the science of Reishi and fast to some method and purpose.

2. Internal Action of Reishi

By the internal action of Reishi is meant the action within the bodily constitution causing all the organs to function. The force of Reishi is thus transmitted to all the matter composing the body, both organic and inorganic, so that all works and moves by vital or spiritual force quite independent of mental or physical action. While the external action of Reishi was at times consciously experienced in the past, the internal action has remained an insolvable mystery, its action manifesting itself only in the erratic or unique. Such experiences as table-turning and other mysterious phenomena are the accidental manifestation of the internal action of Reishi. But these are in no way true examples of the internal working of Reishi, their futility being manifest to all. The proper study of the internal action of Reishi is quite a new problem worked out only by the founder of TAIREIDO.

[97] Hikkei says Usui was inspired to discover Reiki during a period of fasting

The operation of the internal action of Reishi cannot be explained in so many words, but the action is none the less remarkably practical and effective. It is a truth that can be practiced better than explained, and respects deeds more than words. An explanation as far as practicable will be given in these pages, however, since many who read it will not be able to come to the headquarters of the TAIREIDO system for practical instruction. Though all, if present, may practice alike, yet it is realized that all will not read and understand alike. Consequently those who read are earnestly entreated to do so carefully and repeatedly, so as to make no mistakes or false inferences; and then after understanding the science, to practice it faithfully and effectively. Both understanding and practice are easy.

WE believe that *Tairei* is omniscient and omnipresent

Part IV

How to Command the External Action of REISHI

In taking up the study of the science of Reishi the first lesson given is concerned with the preparation essential to acquiring command of the external action of this divine power. These preparations are necessary to all desiring to make any study of the spiritual world.[98] In this system mere concentration of mind or unification of ideas is not regarded as spiritual study and preparation; nor is the mind-suggestion and other tricks of hypnotism admitted to have any relation to spiritual questions. This position is adhered to in spite of the fact that certain possible spiritual phenomena accompany unification of ideas and mental suggestion or concentration of mind. Such coincidences are purely accidental. Spiritual study and culture must involve spiritual action transcending all matter and mind; and the external action of Reishi is emphatically such a study. It is thus quite different from spiritual study as commonly understood in the modern world; and the study of the system of Reishi requires an entirely different

---

[98] As mentioned before, these are similar steps to how many Reiki practitioners engage before treatment.

preparation of body and mind compared with the study of ordinary so-called spiritual subjects.

1. Preparation of Mind

When undertaking a study of the external action of Reishi such tasks or problems as mental concentration, mediums, self-suggestion, auto-hypnotism and attempts at depersonalizing oneself are prohibited. It is fortunate that such trials are not necessary for the study of Reishi, since unification of ideas and mental concentration and all that sort of thing are achievements that even the greatest minds can perform only after long years of practice and struggle. And even if such achievements could be made easy, they would still be no particular help toward acquiring the science of Reishi. Of course while engaged in the study of the external action of Reishi one's mind naturally concentrates and one's ideas naturally unify and harmonize, but such action is quite different from that of devoting one's attention to these acts in oneself. That unification of ideas and concentration of mind that comes from the study of Reishi is natural and not forced, and such a result is to be encouraged rather than discouraged. It is any sort of artificial action of the mind that is to be avoided.

No particular concentration of mind is called for in trying to understand the external action of Reishi. Such knowledge comes from a presentation of the process of Reishi action according to fixed form in a calm and impartial manner. In dealing with science both eloquence and bias are out of place. Eagerness and zeal do many things in this world but they cannot master the science of Reishi. In fact eagerness alone is a hindrance to acquiring this science. Eagerness to learn is, of course, an advantage to the student, but in many cases over eagerness proves an obstacle to progress. One must be patient, cautious and careful so as not to lose the necessary composure of mind; and too strong a desire after mental composure is tantamount to mental disturbance. Consequently the student must not put himself to any mental pains or spiritual excitement, but simply be ready to adopt the fixed form he is taught.

Even meditation, which is so necessary in spiritual exercise, is no particular use in the study of Reishi. In fact it is rather a hindrance, for it demands a concentration of ideas and a state of mental abstraction by which the action of Reishi is prevented. Emotion, feeling, sentiment are violent preventatives of the external action of Reishi! When Reishi acts it does so with vim, and one's body is compelled to do likewise, as the action of Reishi works from its inner source in the body; and this action is so pronounced as to allow no opportunity for meditation, the body being obliged to leap and jump under the stress of spiritual force. It is clear that meditation can be of no use in such a case. This is a matter to keep well in mind. It is not meant, however, that at times when one is not engaged in the study of the external action of Reishi, meditation may not be good, as sometimes it is a very necessary operation in the cultivation of the mind.

In the same way the habit of auto-suggestion is to be rejected as prejudicial to progress in the study of the external action of Reishi. In many cases such condition is not unlikely to exist but it is always to be esteemed a hindrance to any proper presentation of the external action of Reishi. Whatever spiritual phenomena or other result may come during the process of auto-suggestion, all must be taken as the result of Reishi and independent of the means resorted to. Reishi brings about the same experience more effectively in a scientific way. On the whole, however, auto-suggestion is a positive hindrance to spiritual action.

Self-hypnotism is only another form of auto-suggestion, except that the subject becomes drowsy and assumes a sleepy condition. To talk as some do of a hypnotism that does not produce sleep is a self-contradiction in terms and mere nonsense. All the results obtained by hypnotism can be obtained better without it, and if so, they are not really due to hypnotism at all, so that the results accompanying hypnotic action is merely accidental. Thus hypnotism greatly hinders the external action of Reishi. The action of Reishi is anything but quiet or sleepy; it rather wakes one up and gives keen consciousness of living action, the body moving under spiritual force even to a violent degree. Therefore, both the subjects and the objects of hypnotism have to get rid of their old ideas and refrain from all their former practices when they come to study the external action of Reishi.

Finally it may be said that such practices are implied by mental abstraction, or the habit of setting the mind free from all that concerns the visible world, are also a hindrance to a proper study of the external action of Reishi. Certainly the action of Reishi cannot be experienced while one is trying to force the mind into a state of abstraction. Both the willingness to pass into a state of abstraction as well as the state of abstraction is equally obstructive to the study of Reishi. Mental abstraction is not forbidden as a method of mental culture, but it is not to be attempted in connection with Reishi. The external action of Reishi has no connection with cultivation of mind; and as the external action of Reishi is due to oneself any occupation of the mind with other matters must necessarily hinder it. Especially any endeavor to reach a state of mental abstraction will prevent the action of Reishi. Students of the Zen sect of Buddhism, who are prone to regard cultivation of the science of Reishi as another form of acquiring powers of mental abstraction, are especially liable to fall into the error here to be avoided. In studying the external action of Reishi the mind must be calm and free from any effect after abstraction.

If one can keep the mind free from the above hindrances, progress in the study of the external action of Reishi will be rapid and satisfactory. The most desirable attitude of mind for the student of Reishi is one of transcendence of self: keep the mind on this transcendence of self, unrestrained by thoughts of egoism or of one's environment; but if miscellaneous thoughts occur, let them occur naturally without any attempt at coordinating them or concentrating the mind on any of them, not even to the degree of simple meditation, leaving the mind perfectly free to wander its own way. This attitude of mind has a much more profound significance than can be here entered into, but it is not necessary to go into that in order to learn the external action of Reishi. Moreover, in trying to attain the attitude of mind suggested one has to be careful not to fail to attain it by too much anxiety about it. It is sufficient if the mind be kept perfectly free, to feel absolutely no restraint from any cause within or without the mind. Yet if one is thinking how not to be thus restrained one is not in a state of mind to transcend self; and as this state of self-transcendence is necessary, the best way is to be unstrained naturally rather than artificially, when one's condition for learning the external action of Reishi will be perfect.

2. Preparation of the Body

In order to attain proper physical preparation for acquiring knowledge of the external action of Reishi certain fixed forms in sitting and standing are absolute. When the posture is inaccurate, or causes any unnatural physical strain, the realization of the action of Reishi is prevented. To note the natural mode of standing study the illustration. One must not stand simply in a calm manner but in a manner best calculated to bring the mind to a state of self-transcendence. In learning the action of Reishi any unnatural condition of mind or body is prejudicial to good results. For instance, any unnatural strain of the abdomen is not good, since it hinders the external action of Reishi. The muscles of the abdomen must be kept at natural tension, but the power exerted must be natural; otherwise it is injurious to the object desired. All overstrain in such cases is prejudicial to the action of Reishi. Everything must be left to take its natural course.

In setting about acquiring knowledge of the external action of Reishi it is customary to fast for a period and try to acquire the knowledge in the meantime. There is a method also which does not necessitate abstinence. If one desires to learn the action of Reishi without any discipline as fasting and without having proper physical preparation, however, the body is liable to certain physiological action, such as the overstraining of muscles and the overcharging of blood-vessels which hinders the presentation of the action of Reishi. This precaution is more necessary at first, as after one experiences the action of Reishi it is no longer necessary. Then one can present the action of Reishi at will, but one must have the will to make such action present.

Here it must be remarked that presentation of the action of Reishi in the presence of others is absolutely prohibited, as it is much too sacred an action for exhibition. One is free to practice it alone but not in public.

3. Care as to Time

After full preparation for learning the external action of Reishi, mentally and physically, as outlined above, one can very easily learn to present the external action of Reishi by following the accompanying illustrations. But the time for such practice is very important. The very best time for the presentation of the external action of Reishi is between the hours of 1 a.m., and 2 a.m., just a little after midnight. Of course there is no particular objection to practicing in the daytime; but the hours named are by far the best for beginners. When the body takes its proper standing position, closing one's eyes solemnly in the hour of midnight, while all around is sleeping and calm, reciting in silence the prayer: "Zenshin-Tairei, Zenshin-Tairei, Zenshin-Tairei", according to the fixed form, one first finds the finger ends where the hands are clasped, move slightly. The movement, gentle at first, will increase in rapidity and severity until the whole body moves and one springs up even if seated. What a moment of rapture that is! Nothing else in the world is equal to it! At that moment one entirely forgets oneself and one's surroundings, and feels as if Heaven and Earth, God and Man, were ONE: TAIREI and SELF become fused into ONE. Then one is so impressed with the reality of the external action of Reishi, as to be filled with its mystery and thrilled with an experience never to be forgotten.

WE believe that *Tairei* is the perfect unity of the thinking subject and the object thought of, and is the final cause of all the powers of numbers or nullity.

Part V

Acquiring Reishi by Standing Method

1. Correct Position

The student of Reishi has first of all to ascertain the correct position in standing. This means something more than merely standing straight upright: it includes standing correctly in mind as well as body. The body should be erect, the heels together and the toes pointed outward. Then the palm of the right hand should be placed on that of the left hand and both should be laid on the centre of the abdomen, closing the eyes and reciting repeatedly the prayer: Zenshin-Tairei, Zenshin-Tairei, and Zenshin-Tairei! Study the illustration covering this point.

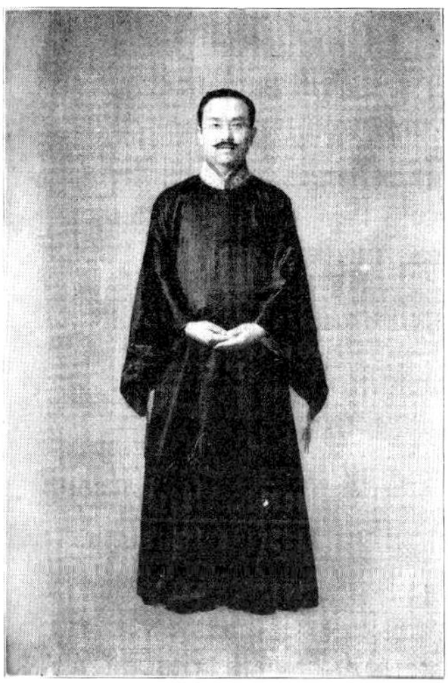

Correct Position
TANAKA MORIHEI

2. Position of Arms

On attaining the correct position in standing bring the muscles of the arms to a natural tension, stretching them down to the very fingers and keeping the latter close together, putting full strength into the palms. Care should be taken to wear no belt and to have nothing on but the lightest clothing, which on no account should be tight. Neither the body nor the mind should be under any kind of constraint. Both should be perfectly at ease so as to act freely. See illustration.

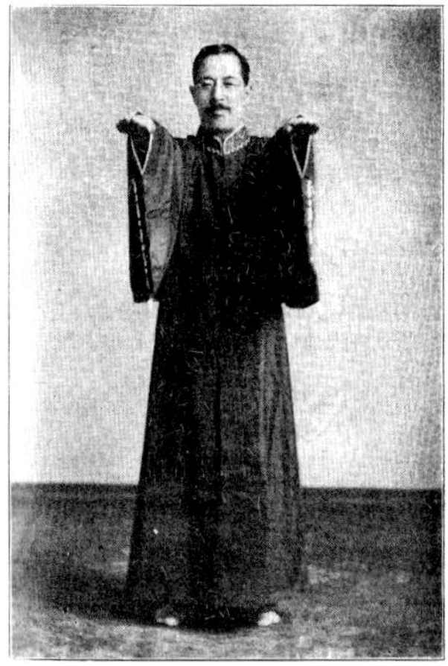

PROPERPOSITION OF ARMS
By Assistant Hasegawa

3. Position of Hands

Before placing the two palms together stretch the arms out fully bringing the muscles to full tension. Then bend the arms without relaxing the strain and join palm to palm, keeping the arms horizontal in front of the body. When the palms are thus together, stress the lower part of the middle finger on the palms, keeping the arms horizontal, and the thumbs some distance from the breast. Then close the eyes and recite the prayer as aforesaid, as shown in the illustration.

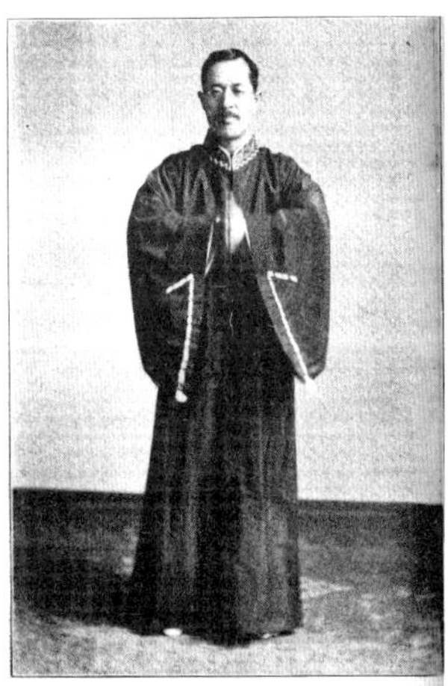

PROPER POSITION OF HANDS
By Assistant Hasegawa

4. Movement of Palms

When the hands are properly joined as above described, the palms begin to move backward and forward. Then give them a chance to move consciously sideways. Instantly there begins a violent side motion. It is quite unconscious motion; yet it is liable to be hindered by leaving the palms wholly to themselves. See illustration 3.

5. Vertical Movement of the Palms

When the sideways movement of the palms becomes extremely violent the palms begin their movement lengthwise. This motion may be produced by conscious action or not without prejudice to the process. But it is very injurious to begin thinking how to produce such motion and why the side motion is changed to a vertical motion and so on. See figure No. 4.

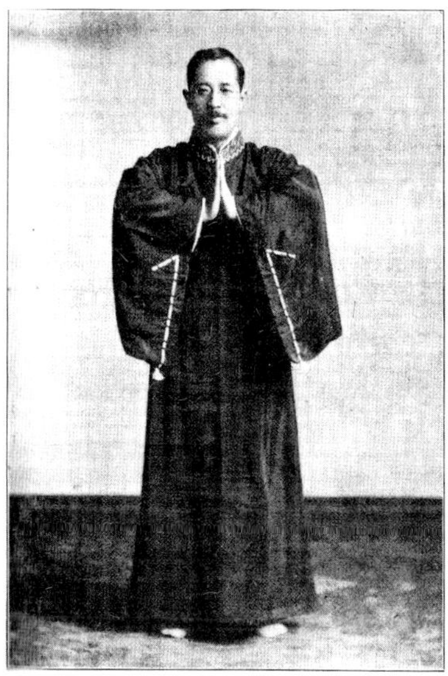

POSITION OF PALMS
By Assistant Hasegawa

6. Movement of the Body

When the vertical motion of the palms becomes very active, the whole body begins moving up and down. Even when sitting, the body will spring up. Finally the body is moving about the room in that state. Then the eyes may be opened. These motions may last only for an instant but sometimes the boy feels as if had been moving from the first. When fully skilled in the practice of Reishi one is quite unconscious of the motions. See figure 5.

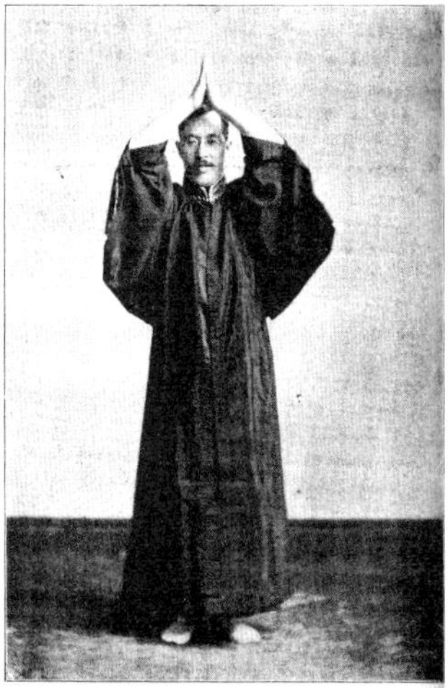

VERTICAL MOVEMENT OF PALMS
By Assistant Hasegawa

MOVEMENT OF BODY
By Founder

7. Clasping Fingers

If preferred one can clasp the fingers but the palms must be kept as close together as possible, otherwise the desired action cannot be expected. But if one attempts to return to merely joining the fingers instead of clasping them no motion will result.

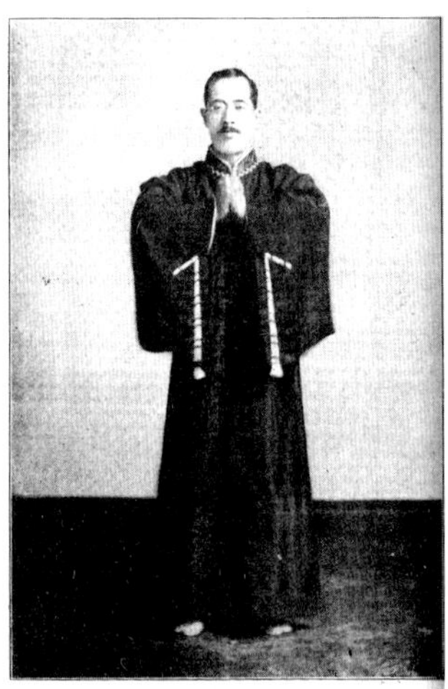

HOW TO CLASP FINGERS
By Assistant Hasegawa

8. Bending Arms and Pressing Palms

When one begins to bend both arms, pressing firmly the palms, the motion of Reishi begins sideways at first and then up and down and finally the whole body moves and springs upward. It is absolutely necessary that these motions shall be left to themselves; otherwise they will not develop. At this time care should be taken to keep the knees quite straight; and this rule must be observed in all cases of standing. In this position the body will spring upward. See illustration.

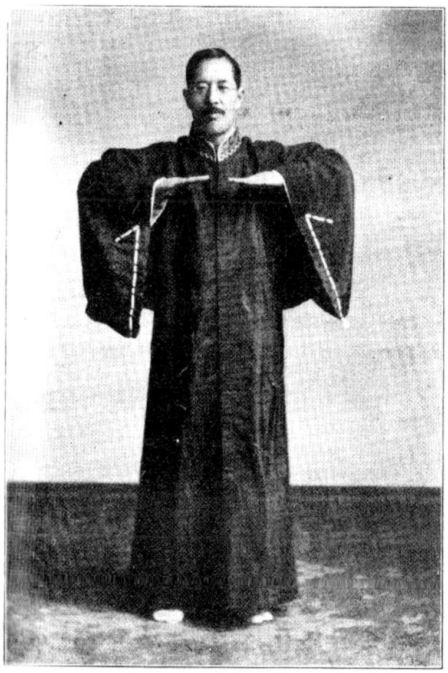

POSITION FCR FRESSURE OF PALMS
By Assistant Hasegawa.

9. Bending Arms While Clasping Hands

By this is meant bending the arms with muscular stress while clasping the hands firmly. In this case, as in simply placing the hand and palms together without clasping, the locking of the fingers and the bending of the arms and the pressing of the palms should be done with the thumbs kept a distance of about one inch or slightly more from the breast. In this case beginners experience certain physiological effects from muscle strain.

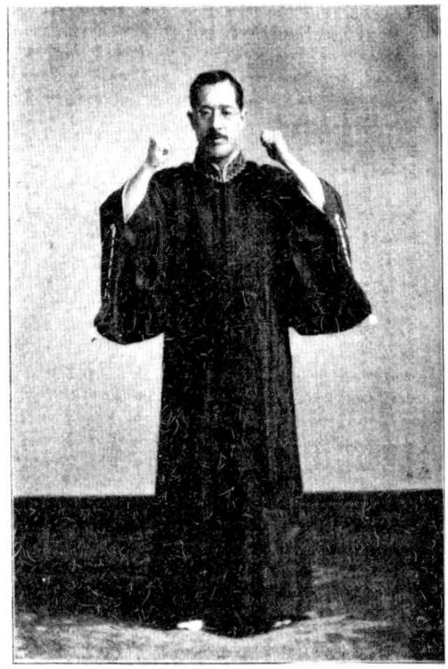

POSITION FOR CLOSED HANDS
By Assistant Hasegawa

10. Stretching the Arms

When stretching the arms, one arm or both may be stretched without the physical operation of stretching the muscles. It is sufficient if one or both arms be stretched out quite straight. If the desired action is not forthcoming one should press the palms more and bend the arms slightly inward. One arm or both may be stretched in front, sideways or obliquely as in figure 9.

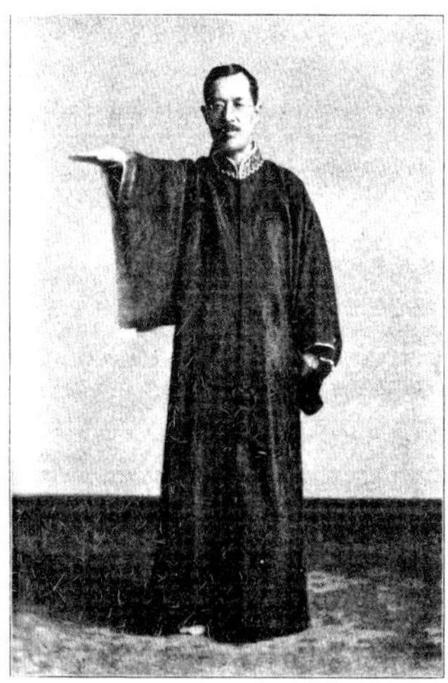

EXTENDING ARM
By Assistant Hasegawa

11. Suspending the Arms

The arms may be allowed to hang without strain, when sometimes the desired action is produced freely and violently. If the action does not come soon the palms should be pressed more firmly or the arms may be given a slight conscious movement so as to lead the action. But it is better to leave the arms to themselves. Then not only the arms but the feet and body also move. See figure 10.

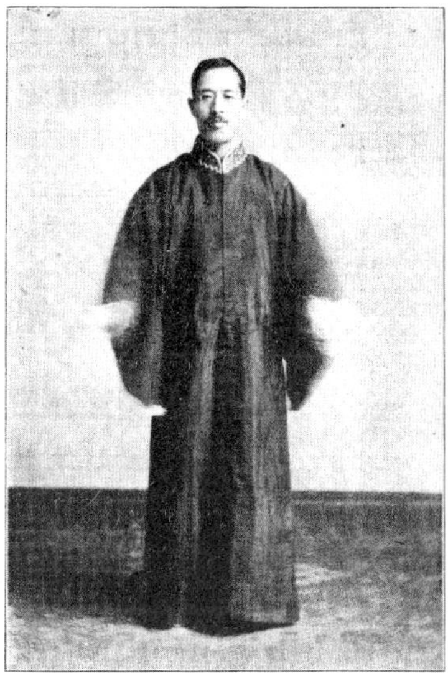

LOWERING ARMS
By Assistant Hasegawa

12. Feet Movement

When the feet move they must be allowed all freedom. One foot or both feet may move without any movement of the arms. When the feet move the body always moves up and down until finally it springs upward. When it springs upward care should be taken not come down on the heels, as a drop of two or three feet on the heels will affect the head. See illustration.

The desired action may be also produced by sitting in a chair or by sitting on the floor and stretching the feet. In this case the action is produced not only in the feet but in one half of the body and sometimes in the whole body. To make the action obtain in the whole body the whole body must be kept quite free and so the posture may be changed at will. The action of Reishi is only for a few minutes in any case.

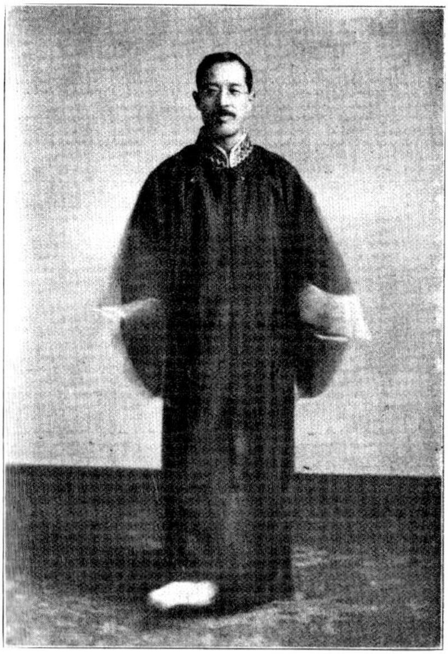

ACTION OF REISHI FEET MOVEMENT
By Assistant Hasegawa

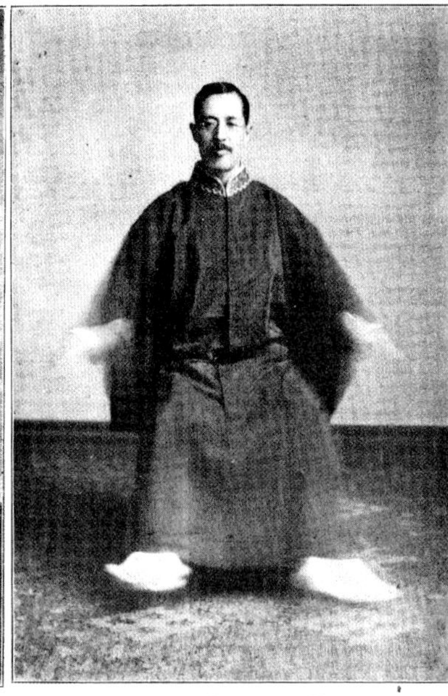

MOVEMENT OF FEET AND HANDS
By Assistant Hasegawa

Part VI

Acquiring Reishi by Recumbent Method

After learning how to acquire Reishi by the standing method one is free to practice the recumbent method. Of the lying down method there are various forms, such as lying on the back or on the breast and raising the feet, stretching the arms and so on. The place, however, has to be very carefully selected. If it be practiced on the bare floor or even on the *tatami* floor it is rather dangerous, as under the action of Reishi the head is apt to strike hard on the floor.

The operation should take place on several lairs of mattresses or blankets piled up; but if only action of the feet and arms be contemplated, protection does not so much matter.

The Spontaneous Method

To be able to produce the action of Reishi in any position, such as standing, lying or any other way, is known as the free or spontaneous method. Even when walking, the feet may experience the action of Reishi. At such moments one walks rapidly as if flying. When the arms alone are under the action of Reishi there is great activity, as if writing shorthand. The experienced one can produce the action of Reishi anywhere at any time: in the hand, the fingers, the nose, and the ears or even in the hair.

Secrets of a Minute's Reishi Action

Any one may learn and practice the methods of Reishi as above explained and directed and thus secure the external action; and such experiences are ideal for promoting good health and good spirits.

RECORDS OF REISHI ACTION

After them the body feels refreshed with great increase of mental and physical energy. That such should be the good result of but a moment's action is unique but true. No other method of exercise or medicine produces any such marked and beneficial result, to say nothing of the great extent of effort and time.

The motion of Reishi involves no less than 720 movements or tremors a minute as a maximum; and no other method possible can produce such motion in the body so quickly and with such exquisite enjoyment. One can easily produce a movement of from 450 to 600 tremors; but one must aim to reach the maximum of 720. As the action is not produced by any outside power there is no experience of weariness or fatigue, but only of refreshment that seems possible only in Paradise.

It is very advisable that the practice of external action of Reishi should take place regularly at fixed times, although any time of day may be chosen. Four times a day are desirable: first in the morning for a minute or so upon rising; the second time for a minute or so just before lunch; the third for a minute or so before dinner in the evening; and the fourth for a little time just before going to bed.

For this any of the forms directed above may be adopted, and the action should be limited strictly to one minute. When this one minute practice is observed regularly and consecutively for a time one will find the mind and body experiencing remarkable development toward unusual health.

How to Measure the Degree of Reishi Action Produced

As already stated the maximum of production is nay one case is 720 tremors per minute. There is a special method by which the number of tremors can be ascertained. One can do this by holding a pencil to paper during the action of Reishi; but this cannot be done for the full time of one minute during which the action lasts. It should be attempted for only five seconds, letting the pencil make waves or dots, like a seismograph. See the illustrations. For five seconds the maximum number is 60, or 12 per second. By multiplying the number produced in five seconds the number per minute can be calculated. For most people the number will be 9 or 10, or about 50 a minute[99].

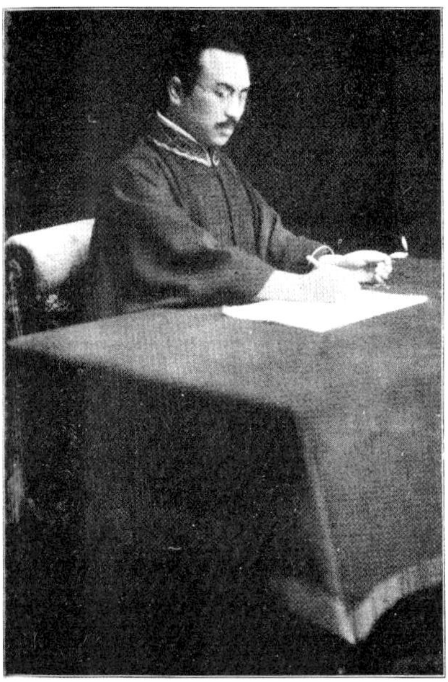

RECORDING REISHI TREMORS
By Founder

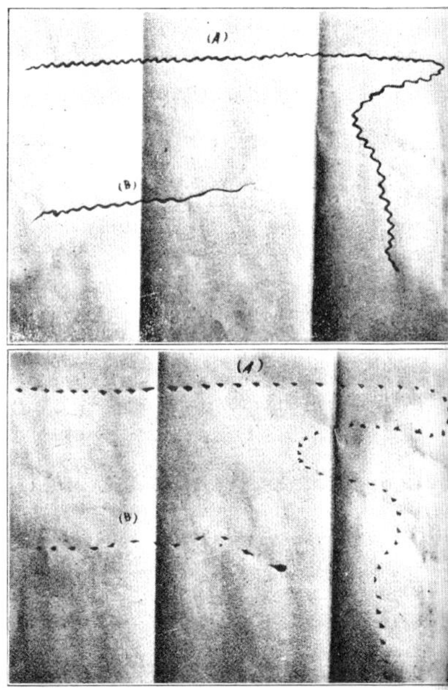

A. Five Seconds Tremors B. One Second Tremors
RECORDS OF REISHI ACTION

[99] It might be interesting for readers to undertake this research

WE believe that everything in the world is rational; and that this rationality has proceeded from the divine will of *Tairei*.

Part VII

Application of Reishi to the Cure of Disease

1. The Meaning

In curing disease in oneself the external action of Reishi is used; but to cure disease in others the internal action of Reishi is necessary. If one has acquired the knowledge and the power to produce the external action of Reishi it is clear that he already has the internal action. When he produces the external action of Reishi to cure some illness the internal action of Reishi within his body grows all the more active and effectual in the cure of the of the disease. External action is, therefore, the chief remedy for Self-treatment. When the external action is produced in the proper way as above directed, with the palms and fingers together there is a joint process of the internal and external action of Reishi working together on the part affected and the cure is certain.

When a practitioner of Reishi comes to treat disease in others his difficulty is to apply the external action in himself to the seat of the disease in others, which is usually internal. Disease in oneself can be cured by connecting the external and internal actions of Reishi in the way described, but how to accomplish this in those ignorant of Reishi is the problem. But one who has acquired the knowledge how to produce the internal action of Reishi can connect the internal and external actions so as to cure disease. Complete recovery, however, is doubtful if only the external action is applied. All cures must depend on the combined working of the internal and external action of Reishi, which can extend their effect to any part of the body, either in self or in the body of another.[100] Such outward affection as skin disease, burns and slight pains, however, can be treated better by the external action of Reishi. Those who possess both the internal and external action of Reishi can bring a cure by external application in most cases.

---

[100] This is a crucial point in the understanding of Tanaka's system.

2. Forms of Self treatment for Disease

The first condition of successful treatment, of course, is to be able to produce the external action of Reishi in the way appointed; and then the application of the action to the part affected. Treatment attempted by application of the hand without producing the external action of Reishi will be fruitless. Violent external action of Reishi is undesirable for healing purposes, just sufficient movement to have the tremor perceptible being sufficient. When the action is too violent the effect is limited to the surface of the skin only. The best effect is to allow a violent motion to begin in the hands which may be restrained to a mild motion and then applied. When a practitioner is unskilled in application of Reishi his hand action will often stop suddenly when it is about to be applied in self-treatment. In such cases the method of bending the arms and clasping the palms firmly should be tried a few times; and then when the external action is again produced without straining the palms in any way, the application can be made and so no cessation of the tremor will be experienced.

3. Four Processes of Application

In self-treatment of disease by the Reishi system there are processes, known as the Pressure Process, the Massage Process, the Strained Palm Process and the Strained Finger Process[101].

(a) Healing by pressure. This process consists in pressing the affected part with the palms of the fingers under the external action of Reishi. The pressure must not be very heavy, but very slight, yet close enough to make a proper application of the fingers to the parts. The palms or the fingers only may be applied according to the size of the affected parts. When the application is made it is necessary to be careful not to separate the palm from the part treated, or to break the connection in any way, keeping the palms close no matter how violent the action of Reishi may be. In use of the palms the whole surface of the palm must be applied to the skin, but in using the fingers it is sufficient to apply the palm of the middle finger. When the space to be treated is a little too large the ring finger may be called into use. In all cases the parts of the fingers to be applied must be the middle joint of the palm. The thumb may be applied too in connection with the fingers where it seems necessary.

---

[101] Usui's Hikkei is almost identical: Pressing with Hands (Pressure Process), Tapping Therapy (Strained Finger), Stroking Therapy (Massage Process)

(b) The Massage Process. By this process the affected part is pressed with the palm of the fingers under the external action of Reishi in the manner of massage. But the movement of massage must not be too strong. The affected part is to be rubbed simply as the natural action of Reishi at the time demands. The process is advisable when the affected part is extensive and the desired affected cannot be expected from mere pressure of the palms or the fingers. The palms or fingers must move over the whole of the affected part. The Reishi action should not be too violent, or else the action will not be transmitted to all the affected part. It will be found necessary, therefore, to restrain the Reishi action as far as possible and leave it a slight tremor in the moving palms of the hands or fingers.

(c) The Strained Palm process. By this process the fingers are pressed tightly together side by side and the whole palm and fingers strained until the external action of Reishi is produced. In this process the palm is not applied directly to the part affected but while under the action of Reishi is held about a quarter of an inch from the part to be treated. The Reishi action is restrained as much as possible; and if the part under treatment is very narrow, care should be taken not to extend the palm beyond the desired part. When the affected part is large the palm under the strain of Reishi should move over the whole part.[102]

(d) The Strained Finger process. By this process the upper portion of the middle finger toward the tip is strained till the action of Reishi is produced and then held about a quarter of an inch or five-eights away from the affected part. If the part is very small care should be taken not to let the finger project beyond the affected part. But when the part to be treated is extensive the finger should move over the entire part. In this process it is very necessary to have the external action fully produced before beginning and to keep it under due restrained during the treatment.

(e) Note: In carrying out the processes mentioned above for self-treatment of disease, the pressing and the massaging processes are the most efficient, and the other two processes should be applied only where the former seem not so well adapted to the treatment.

In the treatment of others the Strained Palm process and the Strained Finger process will be found usually indispensable, but in treating oneself these processes are applicable to only a few ailments.

---

[102] This is how many modern Reiki practitioners may practice today.

WE believe that of a variety of forms of community, mankind is the highest and ultimate.

Part VIII

Application of Reishi to Special Diseases

DISEASES OF THE BRAIN and NERVOUS DISEASES[103]

1. Congestion of the Brain

Congestion of the Brain usually takes one of two forms: congestion of the arteries or of the veins. In the former case the mind is often disordered or even complete unconsciousness is induced. In the latter case the patient frequently suffers from insomnia or feels dizzy or stupid. Under such circumstances it is usually impossible for the patient to treat himself. But if he has acquired the art of Reishi he may be able to prevent such diseases coming on by adopting proper self-treatment in time.

When symptoms of congestion of the brain are felt the patient should apply Reishi by the pressure method with the hands to the whole of the brain region[104]. The pressure should be brought to bear on the temples or the temple and the eyebrows or eyebrow with the middle finger. After that, the forehead should be pressed with the palms, the abdomen should be massaged and from the knee joint to the feet. In this case the palms must be applied directly to the skin.

Patients with congestion of the brain should take care not to apply an ice bag to the brain or pour cold water on the part affected, for that is apt to

---

[103] Doctors may now diagnose or treat some illnesses differently compared to early 1900s. However Tanaka's suggestions for other conditions may still be useful. If in doubt, seek the opinion of a relevant medical doctor!

[104] According to some translations of the Hikkei (e.g. Richard Rivard) Usui said that if brain disease occurs he treats the head.

create a reaction and a rise of fever intensifying congestion. The patient, moreover, should abstain from all stimulants, especially alcohol.

2. Apoplexy

This affection sometimes comes on suddenly without symptoms, and sometimes there is only fainting and at other times simply a state of unconsciousness. If the functions of motion, sensation and reflection be lost, of course, self-treatment is out of the question. If, however, the patient has been a master of the art of Reishi and has been treating himself properly such affection will probably never attack him. It is a case where prevention is better than cure. But one must understand the proper method of treatment. Before apoplexy comes on one is usually hemiplegic, which can be cured by proper application of Reishi action.

The first application should be the pressure of the finger points of the two hands to the temples, the middle finger of the eyebrows, the forehead, the nose side and the ear sides. The pressure process should be applied also to the heart. The whole of the body within reach of the palms should be energetically massaged. In cases of being hemiplegic the massaging process should be applied with rapid movement and considerable pressure to the paralyzed side and still more energetically to the other side of the body, when a cure is certain[105].

The same caution should be observed as in the case off cerebral[106] congestion. Apoplexy is often inherited and those who anticipate it should prepare to avoid it by proper Reishi treatment.

3. Cerebral Anemia

This disease often brings on faintness or insensibility, and sometimes with convulsive effect on the whole body. The convulsive action usually ceases after a little time and seldom ends in death. Congestion of the brain, apoplexy and cerebral anemia are the most dangerous of the brain affections.

The treatment should be the same as for congestion of the brain. It involves the pressure process applied to the whole of the brain region, and especially a strong application of the finger points to the cerebellum, the middle of the

[105] Usui's Hikkei also says that apoplexy can be treated by healing the head area, heart, and paralyzed area.

[106] Usui's Hikkei also puts cerebral palsy with the same heading as apoplexy.

eyebrows, the temples, and the forehead. After that the eyes should be closed and the pressure process applied to the eyes with the finger tips. The abdomen and the feet should be massaged.

All alcoholic stimulants should be avoided. Fomentations applied to the head assist in restoring the circulations of the brain with similarly beneficial results.

4. Nervous Debility[107]

This is an affection found very frequently among the men of the present time; but as yet no very effective remedy has been found for curing it by the medical profession. Numerous medicines are prescribed for it, but none of them has proven effective. The system of Reishi has cured as many cases as the doctors have done[108] and is therefore one of the most satisfactory methods of either prevention or recovery. And it has the advantage of not being attended by the reaction that usually follows the use of medicine[109].

For treatment of this disease the body must first be placed in a proper position. The abdomen should be massaged under the action of Reishi and then covered with the strained palm under the same action. The pressure process should be applied to the cerebellum and then to the entire cerebral region, or the massage process may here be used. Next the pressure process should be applied with the fingers to the temples, and the pressure or massage process to the middle of the eyebrows, the forehead, the eyelids and the sides of the ears. Finally massage the limbs, the breast and the abdomen. Try to excite strength in the muscles of the abdomen. If this treatment be repeated for a few days the trouble will give way in two or three days of treatment, and a serious attack in two or three weeks. If the patient is able to apply the external action of Reishi the cure will come without so much of the above treatment.

The patient must abstain from alcohol, tobacco, stimulants, sexual intercourse and games of all kinds. He should retire early and rise early. He should not be absorbed in reading or writing or anything that causes painful constraint of mind or body.

---

[107] Dr Usui's Hikkei also states Reiki can help nervousness.

[108] Some would argue this is still true today?

[109] The lack of side-effects of Reiki compared to orthodox medicine is shown in many modern research studies. It is interesting Tanaka realized this.

5. Hysteria

Hysteria is another common disease in modern times, and nearly all women are more or less affected with it. It causes a certain degree of mental derangement and sometimes is so extreme as to lean to insensibility. It is brought on by nervous excitement of one kind or another, despair, worry and mental exhaustion. The first step toward cure is to remove the causes of the trouble. If the patient is too far gone to apply self-treatment by the Reishi system then the treatment should be given by others who have mastered the system.

As in the case of treatment for nervous debility, the body should be placed in a right posture. Then the abdomen should be massaged with the palms so as to strengthen the muscles, pressing the carotid artery with the finger tips. Massage the temples also, the middle of the eyebrows, the forehead, the eyelids and the rims of the ears. If a woman's hair is dressed so as to obstruct the treatment the fingers can be pressed into it as far as practicable; for a serious case, however, the hair must be taken down and let loose. As this disease usually produces cold feet they should be energetically massaged, applying the palms directly to the skin.

The patient should abstain from alcohol, and other stimulants; also from tobacco and sexual intercourse. All exciting brooks should be avoided and such duties as needlework, washing and so on. Washing is especially an excitant toward hysteria.

Part IX

Diseases of the Mouth

1. Toothache[110]

Toothache is cured simply by causing the external action of Reishi and pressing the finger tips lightly to the affected part for a few seconds or a few minutes, as the case may require. If pressure is exerted too severely the parts may become blood hot and therefore more painful. The pressure should be exerted from the outside without directly touching the teeth or gums. The ache will decrease gradually under this treatment until finally one can even bite without feeling any discomfort. The more serious the case the longer will be the operation, from 15 minutes usually to half an hour or an hour.

---

[110] Usui's Hikkei mentions healing toothache

It must be borne in mind that if medicine be applied the action of Reishi will have no affect. If the mouth must be cleansed it is better to apply the cleansing after the treatment. It is advisable to be careful as to food; and during treatment it is better to abstain from food.

2. Inflammation of the Mouth

This disease is caused usually by an unsanitary condition of the mouth, or by taking bad milk, addiction to alcohol or tobacco. The causes, therefore, must be removed before treatment begins.

To treat the affection open the mouth half way and apply the stressed finger process directly over the affected part or parts[111], using chiefly the middle and forefinger. The external action of Reishi must be brought on by straining the finger, and direct pressure or massage must be avoided, as it is not advisable to touch the mouth. The discomfort of this affection cannot be removed quickly. Acute attacks will require one or two days, and chronic cases a still longer time.

The effect of the treatment will be realized more quickly if the patient abstain from food for from one to three days, though due care must be taken not to weaken the body, especially in cases of low vitality. The patient should abstain from all stimulants, especially alcohol and tobacco.

3. Cancer of the Tongue

This disease does not occur very often, but when it does appear it is not amenable to medical treatment[112], though it can be cure by the external action of Reishi. For treatment, open the mouth half way, and apply the stressed finger process[113], under which in time the disease will gradually disappear. The finger should not be allowed to come in contact with tongue.

In regard to medicine, food and stimulants the same rules should be observed as in treatment of inflammation of the mouth.

---

[111] Usui's Hikkei suggests to cover mouth with hands without touching lips

[112] Nowadays, this condition can often be helped by orthodox medicine

[113] Usui's Hikkei states that to help tongue, to heal the top and root of tongue

Part X

Diseases of the Throat, Stomach and Intestines

As all animal life is sustained by food this subject becomes one of vital importance, especially to man whose food is of a great variety and, therefore, liable to injure the stomach and intestines. In modern times affections of the stomach and intestines are constantly on the increase; and there is yet no effective medical treatment for such troubles. The Reishi treatment, therefore, is the most satisfactory known, since, if properly applied, it will bring these organs to a natural and healthy condition.

1. Gastritis[114]

In treating gastric catarrh the body should assume an erect attitude, the chest broadened as much as possible, when the fingers should be brought close together and the massage process firmly yet gently brought to bear on the stomach with the finger tips of the two hands, proceeding from above downward. This operation should be continued for a few minutes, after which the abdomen should be massaged with the two palms.

While treating this affection food should be avoided for two or three days. No medicine should be used, as it cannot cure the disease and may greatly complicate it. If medicine must be taken, take one kind only and not a number. Milk and fatty foods should also be avoided, as well as alcohol and all stimulants and drugs.

2. Colic of the Stomach[115]

Produce the external action of Reishi throughout the whole body and then press the stomach firmly with the fingers of both hands. In slight attacks the relief comes in a few minutes, but for a serious case the time required will be some minutes longer. Morphine should not be used, as it only paralyses the stomach and does not remove the cause of the trouble, and the danger of becoming accustomed to such a drug is very great. There is no system so safe or as sure as that of Reishi.

---

[114] Usui's Hikkei mentions the healing of gastro-enteritis

[115] The Usui Hikkei also mentions healing for stomach and abdominal pain

In this as in so many other cases one should abstain from alcohol, tea, tobacco, morphine and all kinds of stimulating food and drink.

3. Enlargement of the Stomach

Press the stomach with the right palm always after eating. Those who can hear a sound of water in the stomach after eating should not drink at meals.

It is very important in this affection to abstain from drinking as far as possible, as liquid aggravates the double [...] (missing text, could be trouble?). Give up soup, milk and other liquid foods and keep to solid and nutritious foods.

4. Tumor of the Stomach

If the patient feels pain after eating the stomach should be pressed with the right palm both before and after meals. The treatment should begin at the first symptom of pain. The treatment should begin at the first symptom of pain. For complete removal of a tumor the stomach must receive the pressure treatment three times a day, morning, afternoon and evening, as well as before and after eating. Care should be taken not to press too strongly.

This is a disease that should be taken seriously, even after it begins to yield to the Reishi treatment. Keep as quiet as possible and be especially careful as to food. Do not drink milk or soup and yet do not take tough food of any kind.

5. Cancer of the Stomach[116]

This disease occurs most frequently in men of between forty and sixty years of age, being seldom found among younger men. Existing medical science can give no reason for the disease and prescribes no remedy. Usually, therefore, when a case is diagnosed as cancer of the stomach the patient is in despair. This is unnecessary when Reishi is ready to affect a cure. The Reishi system can cure a slight cancer in a short time and more serious cases in a long time.

In treating cancer of the stomach the external action of Reishi should be produced in the right palm and applied to the affected part very lightly and gently. When the patient feels pain on pressure of the part, press until the pain is gone. It is injurious to exert pressure too strongly.

---

[116] Usui's Hikkei also mentions the healing of stomach cancer

No medicine should be used; and if medicine must be taken, let it be of one kind only. Abstain from alcohol, tobacco, milk and stimulating foods.

6. Disease of the Gullet

There are various affections of this part of the body, such as stricture, cancer, spasm and so on, all of which can be treated in the same way.

Apply the pressure process to the whole of the gullet and throat at first, and then extend it down to the breast and stomach. Press very lightly, especially in case of cancer.

The patient should abstain from food that is either very hot or very cold, as well as from acid or stimulating food. Alcohol and tobacco should be avoided; and the patient should be kept free from excitement and emotion, being as calm as possible.

7. Intestinal troubles[117]

In case of catarrh of the intestines or constipation[118] massage the entire abdomen with the right or left palm. Then do the stomach, applying the pressure process of the palms to the hips. Use no medicines, but only apply the external action of Reishi so as to invigorate the natural capacity of the body to affect its own cure. The habit of using medicines for bowel complaints is pernicious, especially for constipation, as the trouble is only thereby aggravated beyond cure.

In case of intestinal catarrh one should avoid eating and drinking immoderately, especially decayed or unripe fruit and also water and tea and ice. The patient should fast for two or three days during treatment, if the constitution so permits. In any case do not take milk, which aggravates the disease. The same caution should be observed in regard to constipation.

8. Appendicitis and Kindred Troubles

If the patient feels acute pain and the cecum is swollen the palm should be pressed gently on the affected part, and in a few minutes under the external action of Reishi the pain will be relieved. Even the severest attack will yield to Reishi in between twenty and thirty minutes. As the process is applied repeatedly the swelling will gradually disappear. It is then necessary to

[117] Dr Usui's Hikkei mentions intestine healing.

[118] The Hikkei of Dr Usui mentions healing for constipation.

apply the massage process to the entire abdomen and hips[119], as the disease is liable to cause inflammation in these parts.

Caution as to food is extremely important. One should take vegetable food only, abstaining from fats. Exercise should be very gently; as any sort of violence in this respect is very injurious.

9. Tuberculosis[120] of the Intestines

Though this disease is not very frequent it is very important. Thus far medical science has not successfully dealt with it. It can be cured by Reishi, however, simply by applying the massage process to the whole of the abdomen, treating it three times a day, morning, afternoon and evening, as well as before and after food.

As to food, observe the same precautions as in the case of appendicitis typhlitis.

10. Peritonitis[121]

Apply the massage process very gently with both palms to the entire abdomen, using the pressure process rather strongly on the hips with both palms. Treat further in the same way as for intestinal catarrh. In case of acute pain press the part gently, and relief will be experienced in a few minutes. Continue pressure until the pain is gone.

Do not take much medicine, nor take any milk or potatoes. The same rules of diet as for intestinal catarrh should be observed.

11. Piles

Piles are of different kinds, but all can be treated in the same way by the Reishi system. Under external action apply the finger tips by the pressure process through bandage material to the anus. If the external action of Reishi becomes intermittent during the process, bend the elbows and stress the palms to increase the action and then repeat the pressure process. Haemorrhoidal protrusion does not require any operation as it can be cured completely by application of Reishi.

The patient should abstain from ginger, pepper and all such irritants as well as from alcohol, milk and astringent foods.

---

[119] Usui's Hikkei suggests healing appendicitis via hip, stomach, intestines

[120] In the Hikkei, Usui-sensei mentions healing for tuberculosis

[121] Peritonitis is also mentioned in the Hikkei of Dr Usui.

WE believe that the purpose of a state is to make its members observe order.

Part XI

Various Internal Diseases

1. Consumption, Pleurisy[122] and Bronchial[123] Affections

Up to the present the medical fraternity has found no remedy for tuberculosis of the lungs, so that when one is taken with this usually fatal ailment, the mind is pessimistic and despairing. Yet this disease yields to Reishi as readily as any other, and some of the cures have been nothing short of marvellous. Indeed that a method so apparently simple should accomplish such remarkable results seems almost incredible, were it not known to be true. In cases of pleurisy, too, for which medicine prescribes no sure remedy, the cures have been quite effective, including pleuro-pneumonia[124] which is liable to develop into phthisis, if not properly treated in time. Affections of the bronchial tubes can be removed with equal facility.

In treating consumption the lungs must be pressed by both palms, care being taken not to incite a violent action of Reishi, the most moderate activity being preferable and quite sufficient. The treatment is more effective when the palms are applied directly to the skin instead of through the clothing. The massage process should follow on the breast and pressing process on the larynx. The head should be treated in the same manner as in cases of nervous debility, and the stomach and intestines should receive the same treatment as is prescribed for catarrh of these organs. Medicine should be avoided if possible, as it tends to cause irritation and exhaustion, making the disease worse. The rule as to abstaining from the use of medicine should be observed from the very first. The Reishi treatment should be applied both before and after eating, in the forenoon, the afternoon and at the night, as well as when the patient is rising or asleep, or any time that the attack is most serious. Slight cases can be cured simply by application of the external

[122] Pleurisy are mentioned as a case for healing in Usui's Hikkei

[123] Usui's Hikkei mentions Reiki for bronchitis

[124] Pneumonia is mentioned in Usui's Hikkei for a Reiki treatment

action of Reishi. Be careful to press the abdomen. Ice should not be applied to the affected part to relieve fever, as this makes the matter worse.

For pleurisy and pleuro-pneumonia the treatment is almost wholly similar to the above except that in case of purulence the arms should be brought around to the back so that the pressing process can be applied to the left side of the spine with the palms.

For bronchial treatment apply the pressing process to the larynx and the massage process to the breast.

In the above diseases, especially where the lungs are affected, it is important to avoid alcohol, tobacco, acid foods and such foods as milk, that stimulate the mind and body overmuch. Do not engage in any work requiring attention to details, and avoid bad water and bad air.

2. Diseases of the Heart[125]

For such affection as valve disease of the heart, palpitation, rapid pulse, disease of the aorta or contraction of the heart the Reishi system is most effective. All that is necessary is to apply the pressing process with the palm of the right hand to the heart, being careful not to incite a violent action of Reishi, as that affects the disease adversely. The benefit will be experienced either if the pressing or massaging process be also applied to the head, stomach and bowels.

Ice should never be applied to the heart, as it invites a feverish reaction and may induce rupture of the heart, though there are times when it may be resorted to for a few minutes as a first aid. Abstain from alcohol; and from food that is stimulating or too hot or too cold. A small quantity of wine may be taken if the patient is fond of it.

3. Diseases of the Liver[126]

In affections like hardening of the liver, hypertrophic or congestion of the liver, the Reishi system is always effective, the method being simply to apply the pressing process to the liver with the palms. When pain is acute, as in cases of congestion of the liver, the pressure should be maintained until relief is found. The breast should be massaged down to the abdomen, since the liver affects directly and indirectly the spleen and kidneys as well as pancreas and the lungs.

---

[125] Usui's Hikkei suggests how to help the heart

[126] The Hikkei of Usui also mentions healing for the liver

Alcoholic drinks should be carefully avoided; and any food that is relished may be taken in a moderate degree.

4. The Spleen

Diseases of the spleen sometimes give the skin a dark brownish colour because of derangement in the blood. Vigorous massage should, therefore, be avoided.

5. Diseases of the Kidneys[127]

In all cases of nephritis[128], whether acute or chronic, including dropsy, suppuration, atrophy, inflammation of the pelvis, apply the pressure process firmly to the kidney. When the entire body is affected by dropsy the process should be applied also to the head, ribs and body generally. The pressing process should be applied directly to the pudenda. At the same time the stomach and bowels should be treated as in cases of catarrh of the organs.

A regular quantity of food should be taken, avoiding alcohol, cereals and salty food. The patient should be careful to avoid changes of temperature in summer and winter. No attempt should be made at resistance of the climate.

6. Diabetes[129]

As no effective medical treatment has been found for this ailment it is very satisfactory to know that the Reishi system has proved quite efficacious. The best way is to practice regularly the external action of Reishi, applying the massage process to the lower part of the abdomen and the pressing process to the pudenda. The palms should be moved over the entire surface of the body, vigorously massaging it from the feet upwards. The massage should be against the pores and cover the body as far as the palms can reach. After adequate treatment the urine will become normal and the skin will assume a more elastic consistency. In this way cases that had been declared hopeless, have been completely cured. Special care should be taken of the health, as any second trouble prolongs the disease.

The patient should abstain absolutely from food and drink that contain saccharine matter, including milk and alcohol.

---

[127] The kidneys are mentioned in Usui's Hikkei an area for Reiki healing

[128] Nephritis is mentioned in Usui's Hikkei, for Reiki therapy

[129] Diabetes is also given in Usui's Hikkei. However, it should be noted that it may be dangerous to help diabetics on insulin. For further information, search the Internet or Sweeney's Reiki Level 1 teachings.

WE believe that a state is the only form of organisation through which order and discipline are enforced in the sphere of mankind.

Part XII

Diseases of the Bladder and Generative Organs

1. The Bladder[130]

For such affections as cystitis[131], gallstones[132], spasm or paralysis of the bladder[133], the Reishi process should be applied by pressure and massage to the lower part of the abdomen and then to the urethra. As spasm of the bladder is sometimes accompanied by acute pain it should be treated directly as it occurs. If the spasms be allowed to go on repeating themselves they may become chronic and the cure will be much longer to accomplish.

One should abstain from stimulating food and from alcohol as well as from sexual intercourse, and of anything that taxes body and mind.

2. Hydrocele mention

This trouble usually arises from semen, but is sometimes due to hurt from without. The old remedy of applying an ice bag should be avoided, as it will only intensify the trouble by causing congestion. It is better at first to apply hot fomentations of a degree that will not irritate the skin. But neither medicines nor fomentations are necessary where Reishi is used. Simply the external action of Reishi by the pressing process to the testicles, and soon the fever will abate and the pain be relieved, when the trouble will be cured.

---

130 Bladder stones and related problems are mentioned in Usui's Hikkei

131 Cystitis is given in Usui's Hikkei for Reiki therapy.

132 Usui's Hikkei suggests Reiki can be used for bladder stones.

133 Hikkei cites healing of paralysis can improve bowel movement.

This ailment, which responds to medical treatment so slowly, is quick to respond to Reishi, which at once brings about normal conditions.

While suffering from this aliment and undergoing treatment, it is most important to avoid overwork and all forms of excitement, observing the usual precautions as to food and drink, as prescribed above.

3. Impotence

This affection is caused by a functional change in the penis, brought about by meningitis[134], or sexual excess, masturbation or nervous[135] debility. The affliction should be carefully treated from the very beginning, as, if allowed to develop, it will be attended by various other nervous troubles. First apply the pressing process or the massage process to the lower port of the abdomen, the pressure process to the penis, and the pressure or massage process to the head, stomach and bowels. The external action of Reishi should be practiced and the abdomen regularly stressed.

The lower portion of the abdomen should be dashed with cold water after bathing. Overheated rooms should be avoided.

4. Nocturnal Emission

This ailment is caused by sexual excess, masturbation or encouragement of indecent ideas and the difficulty of incontinence, though sometimes it is induced by such diseases as gonorrhea, prepuce, disease of the spine and nervous debility. The trouble can be cured by practicing the external action of Reishi for a minute or two every night before going to bed.

Every care should be taken not to excite or stimulate the lower part of the abdomen and the pudenda. The patient should also abstain from coffee, tea and alcohol and tobacco.

---

[134] Dr Usui's Hikkei suggest Reiki can be used for meningitis

[135] Again the Hikkei says the same, that Reiki can help nervousness

Part XIII

Diseases of the Motive Organs

1. Articular Rheumatism[136]

Of this affliction there are two kinds, acute and chronic. The application of the external action of Reishi to acute articular rheumatism at once relieves and removes the pain. In chronic cases too the pain can be stopped even with one treatment, but it will return unless the patient receives prolonged treatment according to the seriousness of the case. There are many cases on record where chronic rheumatism of long standing has been completely cured by the operation of Reishi.

In treating articular rheumatism the proper finger should be applied by the pressure process to the part affected; and if the part be large the palms can be applied. If it is a part that can be taken in the hand, it may be seized and so treated. By this process joints which are stiff or painful to move can be easily relieved, the pain almost instantly departing.

Care must be taken to affect a complete cure for the partial treatment and cure leave the disease liable to recur.

2. Muscular Rheumatism[137]

Muscular rheumatism is also acute or chronic. In either case the finger or the palm may be applied to the affected part by the pressure process, by which the trouble can undoubtedly be cured. We have records of many cases where both articular and muscular rheumatism, either chronic or acute, have been completely cured after a short treatment by Reishi. No case of rheumatism should, therefore, be considered hopeless.

In treating muscular rheumatism the same caution should be observed as in treating articular rheumatism.

> WE believe that a state is to exercise the highest authority over its members.

---

[136] Rheumatism is mentioned in Usui's Hikkei.

[137] 'Muscular rheumatism' is specifically mentioned in Dr Usui's Hikkei

Part XIV

Spinal Diseases

1. Myelitis

Myelitis, or inflammation of the spinal cord[138], occurs most frequently from extreme exhaustion, wounds[139], or infectious diseases of an acute nature. To most medical men the affection seems beyond remedy. But it yields to Reishi treatment just as readily as any other disease, especially if the patient receives treatment by the external action of Reishi in the early stages of the trouble. But even chronic cases can be completely cured by proper treatment. The finger should be applied by the pressing process to the spine as far as the fingers can reach, and then the fingers or palms to the ribs.

The patient should avoid cold and heat, preserving the natural temperature of the body as far as possible by the use of proper clothing, blankets or bed clothes.

2. Tabes Dorsalis and Locomotors Ataxia

This ailment is usually divided into three periods, the period of neuralgia[140], the period of irregularity of motion and the period of developing the carbuncle. During the first period the lower extremities are painful, as in cases of neuralgia; and the palm should be pressed over their entire surface, the external action of Reishi being exercised moderately and not to the extent of causing violent motion, such as jumping or springing up. During the period of irregularity of motion the patient is palsied so much that when the eyes are closed as he stands, he is liable to fall or collapse. In this stage the action of Reishi should be applied by the massaging process to the limbs, and the external action of Reishi should be practiced throughout the whole body by clasping the hands together in the proper way, but the action should not be so violent, as to cause spring or jumping. During the last period of the disease the lower extremities are usually paralyzed and it is impossible to walk. Then the massaging process should be applied vigorously to the feet, and the external action of Reishi induced by clasping the hands palm to palm.

---

[138] Usui's Hikkei says to give Reiki for cerebrospinal via the spinal cord.

[139] The Hikkei of Usui-sensei suggests Reiki may help wounds heal

[140] Neuralgia can be helped by Reiki according to Usui's Hikkei

The same caution should be observed as in cases of inflammation of the spinal cord. All spinal troubles can be cured by the application of Reishi according to the method here described.

> WE believe that an individual is an organized form partaking of the nature and power of *Tairei*.

Part XV

Diseases of Women

1. Morning Sickness[141]

In treating this trouble the palm should applied by the pressure method to the uterus, and finally to the stomach, the breast and larynx; after which the pressure or massage process should be applied to the whole head.

During this trouble all acid food should be avoided, as well as that of an astringent quality, and all fats. The patient should also abstain from anxiety and overwork or undue exertion.

2. Endometritis and Irregular Menstruation

Case of inflammation of the lining of the womb cannot be cured usually by surgical operation or treatment. But it invariably yields to Reishi treatment. Cases where the ovary was hardened and enlarged to the size of the patient's fist, accompanied by great pain, were relieved after a few minutes of Reishi treatment, which consisted simply of applying the palms by the pressure method to the part affected. When the external action of Reishi is thus applied repeatedly and regularly the solid is dissolved and the regular process of nature resd, and then the cure is complete.

The patient must abstain from acid and astringent foods as well as fats, and should avoid undue exercise and sexual intercourse.

[141] Usui's Hikkei also suggests Reiki can help morning sickness

Part XVI

Venereal Diseases

1. Syphilis

During the first stage of this disease the pressure process involving the external action of Reishi should be applied to the lower part of the abdomen, and the stressed finger method should be used vigorously on the pudenda. By proper and regular treatment a cure will eventually be affected. For chronic or more serious cases the massage process involving the external action of Reishi should be applied to the entire surface of the body, in addition to the above treatment. The chancre can be cured by applying the Reishi method directly to the affected part. No surgical operation is necessary. If the brain be affected by the malady the pressure or massage process should be applied to the whole head, after the manner described under the head of cases of nervous debility. There are medical remedies prescribed for syphilis, but none of them is quite effective and most of them tend rather to aggravate the disease. The patient must abstain from fatty foods, as they help to extend the ravages of the disease. All use of alcohol should likewise be avoided.

2. Gonorrhea

This disease is considered very difficult if not impossible to cure, as the germ does not respond to medicine. To Reishi, however, it yields readily, though whether the germ is completely eradicated is often a question. The massage process should be applied to the lower part of the abdomen and the pressure method moderately to the pudenda. After systematic treatment in this way the discharge will decrease, and the irritation and pain will depart. Slight cases can thus be cured in a few days and even the most serious in two or three weeks.

Those undergoing treatment must abstain from all use of alcohol, and especially stimulating food which aggravates the disease. Cold also increases the trouble and should be avoided.

WE believe that the life of an
individual is a gift from *Tairei*.

Part XVII

Swelling and Eruptions

1. Carbuncles etc.

Swelling[142] and gatherings can be prevented from coming to a head by applying the pressure method of Reishi to them with the fingers or palms in the early stages of the trouble. If when one part is cured the trouble appears elsewhere the same treatment should be immediately applied and the cure will be affected. If the swelling insists on coming to a head apply the stressed finger process to where the pus is forming. The worst form of carbuncle will yield to this treatment if taken in time.

The patient should abstain from fatty foods, as well as from milk, rice and glutinous food.

2. Scrofula

Some scrofulous erupt from pus while others do not. They more frequently appear on the neck. The pressing finger process should be applied to the part affected. If the treatment be applied early enough no pus will form; but even after it begins to gather, a cure can be affected by proper systematic treatment. No kind of surgical operation or medical treatment can remove the external action of Reishi. After medical treatment the trouble will recur, but not after Reishi treatment.

Abstain as far as possible from all foods containing fat or producing fat.

3. Headache[143]

For a simple headache the head and brain region should be subjected to the pressing or massage process in the proper way, and after being thus treated by the external action of Reishi, relief will be affected. If the headache is serious, repeated treatment may be found necessary. The most effective treatment consists in pressing the finger tips to the temples, and the palms to the forehead. If the feet be chilly massage the soles. The abdomen should be massaged and its natural energy excited. The latter treatment should be repeated until the muscles of the abdomen are strengthened or well developed.

---

[142] Usui's Hikkei suggests swelling will be gone after Reiki.

[143] The Hikkei of Usui mentions headaches as a condition Reiki may help.

Do not wash the head with water or apply ice to it. Bathe the head with warm water instead, or apply warm fomentations. The head should not be allowed to droop or hang down, and all worry and undue thought should be rigidly excluded.

4. Epilepsy[144]

This affliction brings on periods of unconsciousness[145] and sometimes it is accompanied by convulsions. The disease is often hereditary. As it is almost impossible for the patient to treat himself he should see that he has prophylactic treatment. Shock or undue excitement induces an attack and aggravates the disease; so the mind should be kept as far as possible in a state of composure. Those living with the patient should be careful never to display any anxiety about the case, or else the disease will be likely to grow worse.

In self-treatment for epilepsy one should sit in the proper way and close the eyes. Then apply the pressure process to the middle of the eyebrows with the tips of the middle finger, using the right finger first and then the other one, and then all the fingers, touching the temples and finally the nose on both sides, always using only the finger tips. In addition the pressure process should be applied to the cerebellum and down to the cerebrum. Press the larynx and stomach and massage the abdomen. Indeed the whole surface of the body must be massaged, including the limbs, so as to excite a proper circulation of the blood throughout the whole body.

Alcohol should always be avoided, as well as stimulating foods. The patient should not play indoor games of any kind, and should abstain from reading and exciting talk as well as business requiring attention to minute details. The application of water and ice to the head should also be avoided.

5. Neuralgia[146]

There are, of course, various forms of neuralgia, as occurring in various parts of the body. But all can be treated in the same way. In cases of neuralgia of the limbs it is well to avoid using them much or over exercising them in any way. Changes of season often induce exercise of the affected parts should be avoided.

---

144 Epilepsy is a condition also mentioned in Usui's Hikkei

145 The Usui Hikkei suggests ways Reiki may help unconscious-ness

146 It is given in Usui's Hikkei that neuralgia may be helped by Reiki

In treating the disease by the Reishi system apply the external action to the parts where pain is experienced, the finger tips or palms being used, according as the extent of the surface affected requires, the more extensive regions being more amenable to massage process. Acute neuralgic action of Reishi and the most serious cases will yield to repeated treatment. A very serious case may take two or three weeks to cure.

The patient must abstain from alcoholic liquors, and from food containing pepper, ginger and stimulants or irritants of this kind. Undue physical exercise should also be avoided, though the regular exercise of the external action of Reishi is always beneficial.

6. Nervous Prostration or Paralysis

Paralysis of the motor nerves[147] is of two kinds, one involving impotency of nerve function and the other a diminution of nervous force. When Reishi treatment is applied to nerve paralysis in its early stages the effect is usually prompt and effective. If the case be neglected too long it responds to treatment much more slowly. It is only a question of time, however; and if treated properly for a sufficient duration of cure will be affected. In all such cases no time should be lost in applying the treatment. Among the more serious forms of the disease is paralysis of the facial nerves. The treatment for this trouble may be taken as prescribed for all other forms of the ailment.

When suffering from paralysis of the facial nerves press the part with the palms. Usually the trouble is confined to one side of the face only, but the whole face should be massaged in addition to the part affected and where pressure is used. The facial muscles being often similarly affected they also should be subject to the pressure process of the external action of Reishi. Paralysis of the nerves in any part of the body will yield to systematic treatment of Reishi and a cure will be affected.

The patient should avoid the heat of stoves and keep the mind composed and tranquil, as all irritation renders the trouble worse.

WE believe that individuals, including their forefathers and descendants, compose together one system.

[147] Usui's Hikkei mentions nerve pain paralysis

Part XVIII

Insanity

The various diseases of the mind with which a certain portion of mankind is afflicted appear incurable to the medical fraternity up to the present time. Insane asylums have been established in various countries, but these are for the care rather than the cure of those interned in them. If the insane recover in such institutions it is more from accident or nature than from the treatment prescribed or received. There is really no effective remedy for insanity prescribed by the practice of medicine in any country. The reason is but natural, since modern medical science is based on pure materialism and has no remedy for the mind and spirit. On this basis diseases of the mind are treated as affections of material substance and subject to material treatment by medicine, and consequently little or no improvement is affected. Medical science treats man too much as a machine, and the result is that it cures chiefly the material natures. In the region of mind and spirit medical science has affected practically nothing. Indeed it is not too much to say that medicine has aggravated such diseases as insanity rather than improved them in the last few years. The Reishi system views and treats diseases of the mind from quite a different point of view. As our treatment is quite effective we cannot but believe it to be based on truth. We have examples of long derangement of the mind that have been cured by application of the action of Reishi for even a short period.

Of course the self-treatment of mental cases is very difficult, especially if the insanity be complete and permanent. Such cases usually have to be treated by those who understand and practice both the external and internal action of Reishi. Subjected to such treatment all diseases of the mind can be cured by systematic process.

Part XIX

Eyes[148], Ears, Nose and Throat

1. Diseases of the Eye[149]

In treating all affections of the eyes, close the eyes and apply the massage process with the finger tip gently to the surface of the eyelid moving toward the inner corner of the eye and down the side of the nose. Slight cases of such diseases as trachoma can be cured in one or two treatments. Inflammation of the retina or cornea as well as cataract can be treated in the same manner with the same results. The Reishi treatment is especially adaptable to the eye, which is so difficult to treat by medicine and surgery. There are cases where, patients who have been long undergoing medical treatment for their eyes in vain have finally cured themselves by application of Reishi.

The patient should abstain from alcohol and stimulants of all kinds, and should avoid dust and close study.

2. Affections of the Ear[150]

In cases of inflammation or discharge from the ear simply massage all around the ear with the finger tip, and then massage the cerebellum with the palms. If there be no discharge, simply thrust the finger into the ear and transmit the external action of Reishi in that way for two or three minutes, drawing the fingers out abruptly.

Alcoholic drinks and fatty foods should be avoided. The patient should be kept quite and not be allowed to think about the disease, nor be subjected to anxiety of any kind.

3. Diseases of the Nose[151]

For such cases as nasal catarrh subject the cartilage of the nose or the bridge to the pressure process with the finger tip, and then treat the temples in the finger tip, and then treat the temples in the same manner. Finally massage the entire head, more particularly the occipital region, where greater

---

[148] Usui said in the Hikkei that if the eyes are a problem, he treats the eyes.

[149] Usui's Hikkei mentions healing for eyes

[150] The Hikkei of Usui shows how to help the ear canal with Reiki.

[151] Hand positions for nose healing were suggested in Usui's Hikkei

pressure should be exercised. For adenoids the cartilage of the nose should be pressed with the finger tip and all around it as well, when a cure can be affected without resort to surgery. For empyema press the cartilage and environment with the finger tip and massage the parts around the eyebrows. The temples should likewise be massaged and then the whole head. All ailments of the nose can be cured in a similar manner.

It should be remember that although surgical operations are often performed for the removal of adenoids and obstructions of the nasal cavity, the cure is not usually affected, as the obstructions grow again. It is more effective to apply the action of Reishi and remove the irregular action that causes the growth to appear. All who suffer from nasal troubles should avoid impure air as well as stimulants.

4. Diseases of the Throat[152]

Pressure by the right or left palm should be applied to the part affected. Should there be acute pain in the larynx the pressure process applying the external action of Reishi will remove it. Cancer of the throat can also be removed in this way if the treatment be applied in the earlier stages of the disease. Cancer is a disease that is fatal if neglected. It can be cured only if taken before the period for treatment is past.

The patient should abstain from alcohol, tobacco and all forms of stimulating food, as well as from audible use of the voice.

Part XX

Parasites[153]

There are various kinds of parasites, such as round worms, tapeworms, distoma and parasites of the duodenum, which are taken from bad water, raw food, especially vegetables and meals.

In treating the body for such parasites the massage method should be applied with the finger tips of both hands to the stomach, rubbing downward, and then the pressure method with both palms to the whole abdomen. To this method also subject the breast and larynx. The patient should practice the external action of Reishi both before and after treatment.

---

[152] Hand positions suggested to help throat problems are in Usui's Hikkei

[153] Parasites are said to be something that Reiki can help in Usui's Hikkei

If the treatment is properly and systematically carried out the parasites will be discharged from the body.

The patient should avoid taking raw vegetables and meats, as well as raw or unripe fruit and water.

Part XXI

Skin Diseases[154]

In dealing with such diseases as itch, naevus, spots[155] and warts the massage method should be applied to affections which can be touched with the hand and the stressed finger process to those which cannot be so touched. For itch it is better to apply the stressed finger method at first and with vigor, and then the pressure method gently; and a cure will be affected. For naevus the massage method is most effective. Macula, or spots, can be removed by the pressure method. Removal is more difficult after a child has passed the seventh year of age. Warts and enlargements of the skin or glands[156] can be removed best by the massage process, the finger being applied directly.

The patient should abstain from fatty foods and avoid causing the body to perspire.

Part XXII

Wounds[157]

1. Cuts,[158] Contusions and Bruises[159]

For wounds, bruises, contusions and so on, apply the pressure method, or the pain will soon be relieved. The older a bruise is the longer it takes to

[154] Usui's Hikkei mentions that Reiki can help dermatological problems

[155] Usui's Hikkei also mentions spots

[156] Lymph glands are mentioned in Usui's Hikkei too

[157] Information on how to help wounds is in Usui's Hikkei

[158] It is said in Usui's Hikkei that cuts 'will be gone' after Reiki

[159] Usui's Hikkei also suggests bruises can be helped by Reiki

remove it, but if it be painful the distress can be relieved by even one treatment. For cuts, it is better to bandage them if they are large or bleeding overmuch, and then apply the external action of Reishi over the bandage. Both pain and blood will soon stop. For contusion the pressure method should be applied, and relief will soon come. When necessary, and especially when there are many wounds which cannot be all treated in one operation, the treatment should go on for several days.

An immense advantage of the Reishi system is its power to stop bleeding and to heal wounds without resort to surgical treatment.

2. Scalds, Burns[160] and Frostbite

Scalds and burns can best be treated and cured by pressing the palms on the affected part; but if the place be too tender even for this treatment, a better and quicker way is to exercise the external action of Reishi and breathe upon the affected part. It must be remember that the very breath of one having power to exercise the external action of Reishi is quite different from that of ordinary people, and through it the healing power can be conveyed to any affliction to delicate for physical treatment. In this way the pain of scalds and burns can be relieved at once. For frostbite the massage method is best, although the stressed finger or palm may be applied effectively according as conditions suggest.

The patient should avoid all extremes of heat and cold.

3. Bites and Stings

For snake bites, or when bitten by rats or a mad dog, instantly apply the pressure method or the massage method to the affected part or parts. The stressed finger or palm may be used where the conditions so require. For stings and insect bites the same method will bring relief and cure.

It must be remembered that bites and stings though the one takes longer treatment than the other, should be completely cured at one operation. Be careful to see that this is done.

---

[160] Usui's Hikkei mentions healing for burns

WE believe that an individual is the lord of all belongings in the universe

Part XXIII

How to apply the External

Action of Reishi to Life in General

It was suggested at the outset that the action of Reishi is not for curing disease only but a power at the disposal of man for all the purposes of a healthy and wholesome life. Reishi is the source of life, and the proper conduct and action of life depends on it. Its action must accompany every genuine phenomenon of life. Abnormal phenomena or aberrant action of life is not necessarily due to disease, but may be caused by absence of Reishi in full freedom and power. By exercising the external action of Reishi normal action of life can be resd, while constant and regular practice of the external action of Reishi invigorates the natural functions of life and keeps them in a healthy condition, strengthening their resistance to cold and heat[161], increasing natural energy and efficiency, adjusting the body to proper proportions, especially in regard to fat and muscle, making the barren fertile, the person who stammers fluent and so on. The Reishi system may also be applied to military and educational life. Indeed the use of it is coextensive with life itself. It is by Reishi alone that life can be perfected and brought to the ideal for which man naturally craves. How this can be done is outlined in the following pages.

1. How to Resist Cold

On exercising the external action of Reishi one always feels an increase of temperature; and when Reishi is induced vigorously for a minute or two, perspiration will be excited and the body will feel no cold even in the lowest temperature. To one who understands how to wield the external action of Reishi there is no need of artificial heat or wadded garments in winter. A cold wind he welcomes as refreshing. But he has to prepare himself in the external action of Reishi.

[161] Sweeney's classes taught how to endure cold and heat, unless extreme.

The proper way is to get up early in the morning, stand erect, bring the heels together, close the eyes and join the hands, when the external action of Reishi will begin. At first the body moves sideways and then forward and backward and finally it begins to spring or tremble until the number of times reaches between fifty and one hundred. After that one should breathe hard, taking long breaths, stressing the abdomen, grasping or clasping the fingers firmly and pressing the abdomen. At the same time the soles of the feet should be strained or stressed, bending them inward toward one another. Then again induce the external action of Reishi slightly for a few minutes, so moderately as not to re-induce the springing motion of the body.

The temperature of the body is not something that can be reckoned in quantity, as the medical practitioners teach: it is produced by means of Reishi. It is usually explained as the result of hydrocarbon combustion caused by friction of the blood passing through the blood vessels. But the real truth of the matter is that it is due to the action of Reishi. When the external action of Reishi is induced, the natural result is a rise in the temperature of the body. If one induces the external action of Reishi before taking a cold bath he will find only the utmost refreshment. Some people impair their health by bathing in cold water under low temperature, but if they exercise the action of Reishi such a bath will prove harmless if not beneficial. The soldier exposed to extremes of temperature on a forced March can plunge thorough the blizzard or even into icy stream without injury, if he knows how to exercise the action of Reishi. In the same way he can prevent death from frost. The mariner exposed to the dangers of the sea can preserve life in icy water by inducing the action of Reishi.

To inure the body to cold, the practice of the external action of Reishi should not be limited to the time of getting up in the morning; but it should be repeated at any time convenient, preferably, again in the afternoon and evening, a few times on each occasion.

2. How to Endure Heat

The practice of Reishi is an excellent way of becoming immune to the untoward effects of extremely high temperature. By the power of Reishi one can become equally immune to the bad effects of either heat or cold. One simply has to understand how to accumulate sufficient power of resistance. It is a power that can be cultivated only through the use of the external action of Reishi. On one occasion a certain foreigner expressed astonishment at the indifference of certain Japanese to extremes of temperature, and said that the Japanese must have a constitution like asbestos. He also expressed the opinion that the superiority of the Japanese armies in the Russo-Japanese war was due to this power of endurance in low temperature. But when this foreigner entered a Japanese bath and found the temperature too high for him to endure even a moment, he averred that the Japanese must be composed of some insoluble or inorganic substance, as the baths used by the people would scald a foreigner to death. This asbestos quality of the Japanese constitution, which is not seriously effected by either extreme heat or extreme cold, is only an example of our native power of resistance. But however one may be equipped naturally for resistance of heat or cold, the practice of the external action of Reishi is the only sure way of securing this power for all.

To cultivate resistance to extreme heat one should induce the external action of Reishi in the usual manner, at any time of the day or night, as occasion demands, the operation being confined to a minute's duration at a time. After the operation one will feel a rise of temperature and perspire freely, but soon a normal temperature will return and one will experience a feeling of real refreshment.

Soldiers on the March in the heat of summer will find the Reishi method the best way to inure them to the blazing sun and so avoid sunstroke. The latter trouble occurs usually through abnormal increase of perspiration, lessening blood humidity and dulling the action of the cells. And so sunstroke can be prevented only by offering some compensation for this loss of humidity. By the practice of Reishi the humidity is lessened through perspiration before one starts on the March and gradually gets into a state of self recovery by the time the march is under way. Reishi action naturally adjusts all the conditions of life. As Reishi action is the natural cause of temperature in the body it is also the natural restorant of conditions affecting temperature, including the necessary humidity of the blood. Not the temperature of the body and not the humidity of the blood are matters of quantity that can be measured, as doctors aver, but are products of the action of Reishi. All men, whether soldiers or others can apply the action of Reishi to res proper temperature whether of heat or cold.

3. Restoration of Energy by Reishi

Energy is the source of all human activity. There can be no motion and no working without it. A dangerous feature of the modern age is lack of energy, owing to overexertion in the struggle for existence. Energy must, therefore, be increased in proportion to the amount consumed. Yet no adequate means has been found by science for the supply of exhausted energy. Athletic exercise, wrestling, boxing and other artificial means have been employed to res energy to weary bodies, but the fact is such means tend to waste energy! In a busy age like the present man naturally desires to get as much benefit as possible in the briefest space of time. A maximum of good at a minimum of expense is his motto. But the artificial methods mentioned require more time and energy than they compensate for. They cannot be really trusted to res the energy man needs for his daily task.

For restoration of exhausted or wasted energy Reishi is the ideal method. It requires a minimum of time and is always effective. It is a way to everyone, old or young, man or woman, rich or poor. All that one has to do is to induce the external action of Reishi for a minute, or even only a few seconds, before going to work. After such practice it will be found that no work will bring fatigue. If one feels exhausted from overexertion or other causes, let the external action of Reishi be induced and the tired feeling will pass off and one can go on working, even for then hours a day, without experiencing any ill effect. Reishi not only ress but prevents loss of energy.

4. How to Promote Animation

As has been already said, energy is the secret of success in all human achievement. Without it nothing great can be done. Now no one can say he is in possession of full energy unless he enjoys good spirit, and commands a natural degree of animation. It is possible to be energetic without being high-spirited. Abundance of energy is a matter of the body but animation is a matter of the mind.

To animate the spirit by the Reishi system all one has to do is to practice the external action systematically and regularly. This gives one such strength and command of spirit that one has a powerful influence over the minds of others. If we are anxious to influence another toward a certain decision which we believe right, we should practice the external action of Reishi before the interview. In interviews and all forms of negotiation the previous practice of Reishi will give one an attitude of great confidence and advantage which cannot fail to be imposing and impressive. A regiment or an army going into battle under the influence of Reishi will feel invincible and fearless and will surely win. In general struggle for existence, as well as in all matters of difficulty in daily life, Reishi can make one victorious.

5. Reishi makes one Eloquent in Speech

It is hardly necessary to say that much of one's success in life depends on being able to convey thought accurately to the minds of others. This depends on one's command of words. But there is no practical rule for the requirement of eloquence or impressiveness of speech. The methods prescribed are difficult to learn and very uncertain in result. By faithfully practicing the Reishi method one becomes convincing in the best of all ways, namely, by convincing the reason and influencing the will. There is a difference between pleasant speaking and persuasive speaking. There are many pleasing speakers but very few convincing ones. Men often speak with great fluency but with little or no effect. Their speech lacks strength and dignity, and the hearers are unmoved. On the other hand we sometimes hear a speaker without such show of eloquence who nevertheless moves his hearers to action.

When one specially desires to make an effective speech he should practice the external action of Reishi until he has acquired a masterful spirit and personality. He requires both energy and spirit. His position of body should be erect and the strength of the abdominal muscles must be increased. The external action of Reishi should be more particularly practiced on the tongue. This is done by keeping the mouth half open and beginning the external action of Reishi with the middle finger tip at the root of the tongue, working toward the tip. If one has learned how to produce the external action of Reishi in the members of the body the action can be readily produced in the tongue without resort to the use of the finger. The action should be of unbroken duration and the best time for it is just before going to bed at night. The action should not be practiced in the presence of others. It is good to practice it just before making a public speech. During the practice of the external action of Reishi in the tongue the latter should not be protruded from the mouth, for if this is done the lips and jaws will produce the external action of Reishi and deprive the tongue of the benefit intended. The application of the external action of Reishi to stammering and other defects of the speaking organs is equally effective.

6. To Promote Efficiency

Some men are naturally efficient and some are not. But the man of meager talents can acquire great efficiency by the diligent practice of Reishi. As the success of all enterprise depends on Reishi the acquirement of efficiency likewise can come only from the practice of this system. To promote efficiency, in addition to the regular practice of Reishi, the external action should be exerted with the palms by pressing the whole head for a minute or so four times a day: morning, noon, evening and later at night, after which, if regularly and systematically done, one will feel a remarkable increase of mental and physical efficiency. This will be found true of all ages, old or young, men or women, who, if they diligently practice the external action of Reishi, will not only improve their own efficiency but that of mankind as well, since efficiency is contagious. The more mediocre one us the more one has need of Reishi; and those who are unduly defective have need to practice the external action of Reishi in the same manner as the prescribed for nervous debility and inflammation of the intestines, including applications of the treatment to the age of seven years than afterwards. Up until the age of fourteen, however, a cure is more or less easily effected; but just before and immediately after the age of twenty-one, is the most difficult period to cure this affection. This means that the earlier one resorts to the practice of Reishi for the cure of mental indolence and stupidity the more likelihood is there of a speedy cure. The practice of Reishi in the manner and for the purpose described will be found particularly effective in bringing those of common ability to attainment and those of unusually meager ability up to the average ability.

7. How to Grow Fat [162]or Thin

It is, of course, as bad to be too fat as too thin. Every man should aim to keep his body of normal proportions. Sometimes increase of flesh or loss thereof is due to disease; and if so, the disease should be cure before attending to question of one's size. In any case the normal state of the body can be resd by the practice of the external action of Reishi, which regulates the normal action of physical functions. The action of Reishi is producing normal action of one's bodily functions is quite independent of food. Obesity is believed to be due to eating too much fat and leanness to eating too much vegetable food; but Reishi will keep the body normal size no matter what food one eats.

All that is necessary is to practice the external action of Reishi about thirty minutes before each meal. It is necessary to emphasize the necessity of inducing the action before eating, as, if done after a meal, it produces an abnormal condition that may adversely affect the stomach and bowls. Reishi should be practiced not less than thirty minutes before eating. Then after the meal the stomach can be massaged with the tips of the fingers, from above downward, and the intestines should be pressed with the palms. If these directions are carefully carried out, the normal functions of the body will be so regulated as to produce only normal proportions physically. The body will be neither too fat nor too thin.

---

[162] Fat (and obesity) are mentioned in Usui's Hikkei

8. Inducing Conception

When conception does not occur it is usually due to some affection of the uterus[163] or ovaries, whether malformation or disease; and the trouble, when ascertained, should be cured by proper application of the action of Reishi, after which conception will be made possible. This method has been found effective where the most powerful medicine prescribed by doctors had no effect, and even where surgical treatment had been tried in vain. Barrenness, however, is often the fault of the man, rather than of the woman, due to disease of some kind, such as hydrocele or gonorrhea. In either case the practice of the external action of Reishi will bring about normal condition of the body and produce fertility. There is much else that should be said in this connection, but it is not esteemed advisable for publication, being a matter rather for consultation.

9. Reishi for Military Purposes

In a preceding paragraph one or two ways were indicated in which the practice of Reishi could be of great advantage to the soldier and military officer. Soldiers who practice the external action of Reishi regularly and systematically are naturally full of energy and the best fighting spirit, as their physical constitution is first of all improved and then their animation is always up to standard. Not only, so, but their power of reasoning and perception as well as their memory and strength of will are improved and developed, by which military efficiency is greatly promoted. When soldiers are well and cheerful and intelligent they never shrink from danger, whether of climate or battle.

Let the soldier or military officer practice the external action of Reishi for a minute or two every morning when he gets up and before going to bed at night, and he will find a remarkable improvement in his body and mind. He will experience still greater benefit if he also practices it about thirty minutes before eating and about thirty minutes after his meals, preferably after lunch and supper. At the time of the operation he should not wear boots, which will prevent the springing motion.

In time of war and especially during action the stretcher bearers and the ambulance corps should know how to apply the method of Reishi to their patients; as well as to themselves, so as to keep in the pink of condition. The aviator, too, should learn to practice the external action of Reishi, as the best way of developing all his mental and physical functions and keeping them

---

[163] Usui's Hikkei mentions uterus healing

in perfect condition. Such practice would save many an airman from the mistakes that lead to disaster. As the practice of Reishi makes the most dull-witted man efficient and the bright fellow more so, it cannot but be of great use to those entrusted with the responsibility of navigating the air. Were the practice of Reishi general among aviators there is no doubt that the air service would become not only more efficient but see a much more remarkable development.

The same may be said of the men who manage the submarine. Reishi enables a man to meet all circumstances with fortitude, since it keeps his functions and faculties in normal working order. It helps him to hold his breath and be capable even when plunged under water. It makes keen his senses so as to perceive the nearness of danger, and enables him to have the presence of mind to know how to deal with it. There is no doubt that in all future wars the issue will be decided by those in control of the air and the ocean. Consequently nothing could be better than to have all Flying Corps and Submarine officers and men practice the Reishi system.

It is now clear that the wars of the future cannot be won simply by having plenty of soldiers and enough money to finance them. Success will depend most of all on the efficiency of the guiding and fighting personnel. One can have no doubt that the most efficient fighting army of the future will be the army making the largest use of the Reishi system.

10. Reishi in Education

There is no doubt that the education of today is too much based on materialistic notions and mechanical processes that restrict the natural freedom of developing minds and bodies. The natural talent of the individual is curbed and stunted rather than developed and sharpened. The people are already much dissatisfied and there are signs of revolt against so unnatural a system. Men everywhere are seeking freedom of spirit and vigor of mind and body as the best inducement to education. Such is the demand of all the most intelligent minds; but as yet no one seems to have found a way to meet it. To minds and bodies thus in need, TAIREIDO comes with sure relief. This new way of thought and action has brought to thousands[164] in Japan a new light on life's way and a new power to follow the true way, dissipating all former bewilderment and indicating the true method of education. All education in future must be based on TAIREIDO. The fundamental principles of this new thought have been set forth elsewhere,

[164] If Taireido helped 1000s, Usui-sensei almost certainly heard of it

and all that one need do here is to show the application of these principles to the education of man.

As already indicated the action of Reishi is the source of all life and spirit and matter, whence issue all living phenomena. The application of this power to the mind and body cures all irregularity in them, as a negative action; and increases their efficiency, as a positive action. Every desirable change in the phenomena of life can come and will come from the application of the action of Reishi. In no sphere can Reishi be more profitably employed than in giving youth that vigor of body and mind necessary to produce great manhood and womanhood.

Boys and girls should all be taught the practice of the external action of Reishi; and especially in school they should be obliged to practice it after every gymnastic exercise or drill. The external action of Reishi is especially easy for young persons to induce; and when they thus begin early and continue to practice it regularly in a systematic manner through life the power of Reishi naturally attains a marvellous degree of development in them, producing minds and bodies of perfect faculty and uncommon vigor. Under the power of Reishi every function of the body and mind will develop normally and the mind will be efficient in the acquirement of knowledge and its application. Reishi is for every grade of school, from primary upwards. As already suggested, those who begin it earliest will attain the greatest expertness in its use. But it can be commenced any time. It's always better late than never. If the practice of Reishi be introduced into high schools and universities a great improvement will soon be experienced in the reasoning and retentive faculties of the students. Imagination will increase and strengthen; powers of comparison, discrimination and invention will be more pronounced; judgment and capacity for analysis and synthesis will show wonderful development.

The Art of Reishi in Outline

TAIREIDO preaches no empty theories nor indulges in vain illusion. Its aim is to apply true thought and theory to actual life, enabling man to realize truth effectively and convincingly in his actual experience. One has only to perceive accurately the truth of the universe in order to see the significance of human life and secure the principles that make the mind at peace. These scientific principles one realizes in practice by means of the Art of Reishi. Only thereby can man enjoy complete development of mind and body and thus enhance the progress of life and the joy of existence. TAIREIDO thus leaves nothing to be desired in its illumination of human thought and life, either in theory or application.

The art of REISHI means the application of the fundamental principles and substance of the universal life to the perfection of human existence. It not only supplies the key to life's significance but to the miracles and wonders that life displays. When the Action of Reishi is applied to human life, whether mentally or physical, the effects are more marvellous and more real than anything recorded in the annals of miraculous cures, and more amazing than the outmost that man has dreamed of in the past. The Art of Reishi can be easily acquired in a scientific manner by any one who desires to understand it; and every one who understands it can apply it and practice it at will.[165]

1. The Action of Reishi

The Art of Reishi involves certain formulae for inducing the action of the fundamental substance or essence of life and for its proper and effective application to the needs of man. It has already been explained elsewhere how Reishi is the primal cause of all existence, whether physical or spiritual, the very essence of all life; but the proofs of this can be seen only by understanding the Art of Reishi. The practice of the Art of Reishi produces wonders nothing short of miraculous in the human body. These amazing results are not due to mental or physical action, but to the operation of the divine principles on which wholesome existence depends. Though produced in the sphere of the material or spiritual or both, they are not the result of physical or spiritual action, but due to the action of Reishi, the Essence of all that is fundamental in material and spiritual existence.

The Art of Reishi involves two actions, the one External and the other Internal.

The External Action of Reishi

The External Action of Reishi means the appearance, on the surface of the human body, of the Action of Reishi as the result of obeying the laws of its induction. When the External Action of Reishi is induced certain marvellous phenomena are observed. At the moment of the appearance of the External Action of Reishi the body experiences a tremor amounting almost to violence, the action being wholly automatic. The movement is slow at first, especially in the early stages of one's knowledge of the Art of Reishi, but increases with experience until the degree is one of considerable vigor or even violence. The relief from all bodily ailments and the general

[165] Usui gives almost the same statements in his explanation of Reiki Therapy in the '*Hikkei*'

refreshment of mind that one experiences at the moment of the External Action of Reishi is beyond the conception of those ignorant of the Art. It is, however, within the reach of all who acquire the Art of Reishi, and is capable of removing all physical and mental ills.

The Internal Action of Reishi

The Internal Action of Reishi means the process of sending the External Action of Reishi, after it appears on the surface of the body, into the body so as to reach any or all parts thereof, as well as the transmission of the Reishi Action to the bodies of others, whether of animals or human beings. The point of contact for transmission is the palm of the hand, especially when the action is to be transmitted to animal or man. It is a power that can be transmitted through any distance, and be made to influence the mind of individuals anywhere at the will of the practitioner. The Action of Reishi can also be used to communicate with others as well as ascertain distant information. Indeed the entire list of phenomena that can be produced by the Action of Reishi would be impossible to explain in mere words. Action of Reishi would be impossible to explain in mere words.[166]

2. Application of the Action of Reishi

The Art of Reishi, involving the underlying principles of all existence, is very extensive in its application. The most beneficial application of the Art is in the way of healing disease and freeing the human body from all forms of evil that afflict it. Notwithstanding the progress of modern medical science there are many ailments and diseases still beyond its power to remove. For this reason there have arisen practitioners of spiritual and mental remedies for the cure of bodily affliction, none of which are quite successful in accomplishment of what they profess to do. But the Art of Reishi requires no medicine[167] and needs no apparatus[168], and yet it performs all that it promises[169]. Independently of the faith of the patient[170] the practitioner of the Art of Reishi can transmit the healing power to the part affected. The practice of the Art is as simple as it is free from danger. Yet it is absolutely efficacious in its results. It is the ideal form of treatment

---

[166] Usui-sensei also found it difficult to explain this in words.

[167] Usui's Hikkei: 'There is no need for the patient to take bitter medicine.'

[168] Usui's Hikkei says: Reiki 'never avails itself of medical equipment.'

[169] In Hikkei, Usui says, 'and in a short time the said diseases will be cured.'

[170] Usui uses similar language in the Hikkei: Reiki 'Does not require consent of patient or any loyalty to the practitioner.'

just because it is the operation of the law on which all life depends. Its effective action on persons distant from the practitioner is especially wonderful and quite effective. Numerous cases of chronic affliction and disease have been cured by Reishi. Nothing can be more beneficial to mankind than to diffuse the knowledge of Reishi as widely as possible.

In so brief an outline as this the theory of the effects of the Action of Reishi on various diseases cannot be fully dealt with. But this is treated in detail in the volume on TAIREIDO[171]. Suffice it to say here that when the Art of Reishi is practiced on oneself or on others, its healing qualities are so manifest as to need no further proof. It sets free the natural capacity of every living thing to operate according to the laws of true life. This natural capacity of the living body to res its wounds and other interruptions of the laws of life the Art of Reishi intensifies to the point of invincibility, ensuring a cure, whether the disease is external or internal. The efforts of medicine are clearly no more than attempts to lead or induce this natural capacity of the body to return to its normal condition; but the Action of Reishi is the body asserting its natural capacity to res any interruption of its process in a perfect manner that only the Art of Reishi can induce and teach. In fact there is nothing that can ail either the exterior or the interior of the human body that cannot be cured by the Action of Reishi. When the Action of Reishi is induced on the exterior of the body the essential principles on which life depends are set free to act without restriction in restoring the interrupted functions of the mind or body. This is more natural and effective means of healing than any other. Some may doubt the possibility of applying the Art of Reishi at a distance, but it is no more impossible than wireless telegraphy or the wireless telephone. Of course the principles are different from those of wireless communication, but yet just as practical in operation. If there is a world which transcends the world we know, there can be no doubt that the laws on which life depends not only exist but transcend all that interferes with the normal action of life, and therefore can be brought into operation for the relief of all human affliction.

It would be a mistake, however, to suppose that the Art of Reishi is chiefly for the diseased and the afflicted. Even for the healthiest of men this knowledge is essential to a proper understanding of life and how to keep its functions in proper order. The daily practice of the Art of Reishi assists the body toward full development of its potential capacity and brings the individual to full bloom of his powers. At the same time it is the only sure

---

[171] This book includes both volumes that were published in Japan in 1916, and is probably the translation of the 1910 volume.

preventative of disease. The Art of Reishi is essential for the development of body and mind and for preservation of health in every way. Only a few minutes a day are required for practicing effectively the Art of Reishi. No matter how robust one is, the wear and tear of daily existence is sure to tell against permanence of perfect functioning of the physical machinery. It is only by applying to the ageing functions this Art of Life that one can maintain health through all experiences, and res it after it has been lost. No one has a command of perfect health and spirit every day or at all times; but knowledge of the Art of Reishi can secure this immense advantage to man. To be relieved from the present dependence on physicians, medicines and pabulums of all kinds for the rendering of existence more endurable is a boon with which nothing else can be compared. At the same time the Art of Reishi is found a most effective means of improving education, military conditions, household matters and everything that pertains to the proper working of human life and civilization. Reishi involves the fundamental laws on which all perfection of life depends.

3. Is a Perfect World Impossible?

As one faces the innumerable ills of life the idea of a perfect world seems nothing but the wildest dreams. To one who understands TAIREIDO and has acquired the Art of Reishi a perfect world seems not only possible but bound to come as soon as man understands and obeys the law of true existence. Mankind will not act aright until the world thinks aright; and this mankind will not do until the principles upon which life functions are understood and practiced. TAIREIDO teaches these principles both in theory and application. TAIREIDO is, therefore, a summons to the peoples of the world to come to the true Light and be led to life. Only by following this Light will mankind come to its divine heritage!

TAIREIDO

1. [172]The doctrine and teaching of TAIREIDO embrace the whole nature of TAIREI, or the Supreme Spirit, and lead the mind to attainment of complete truth, growth and perfection.

---

[172] These seven Principles of Taireido are repeated towards the end of this book, without numbering, and using very similar language, as part of an article published by The Japan Magazine in December 1918

2. The system of TAIREIDO embraces and yet transcends all Religion, Philosophy, Science and Ethics. TAIREIDO exhausts the truth of the universe, and defines the true meaning of human life.

3. The object of TAIREIDO is to unify human thought and bring mankind into closer kinship.

4. Taireido brings peace to the mind of man, and therefore peace to the world.

5. Taireido gives perfect health of body to man and so to the whole world.

6. Taireido reveals the true foundation of Society and the basis of national life for all mankind.

7. Taireido develops and perfects the intellectual faculties of man and reconstructs human life on an eternal foundation.

A Message for Mankind

[173]As one surveys the world today it is clear that the greater portion of mankind has lost the real significance of existence and fails to recognise the true value of human life. There is much physical and intellectual toil and yet no finding of the path that leads to true life. Mankind lacks a true centre of thought, and has no conception of the absolute nature of things and therefore no respect or reverence for truth and reality. The wandering mind of man is thus at sea as to what to depend upon, and life for most people is unceasing bewilderment. No one can truly affirm that mankind today is in a line with truth. In spite of the universal eager haste for satisfaction of human instincts, there is no real reflection, no perception of inspiration. If this process continues human society can only descend to disintegration and ruin. The war in Europe is only a trifle compared with what awaits mankind ignorant of its true destiny[174]. Even without such cataclysms humanity will come to ruin simply for want of capacity for introspection. The war has its appointed end, but the fatal lack of introspection goes on.

It is man's custom to talk of his progress and to boast of modern enlightenment, but it is evident that human society as yet has not reached a stage beyond mere mass or substance. To thrill this human mass with real life and penetrate it with absolute thought is the only hope of man to be

[173] Much of this section of the book is still relevant today.

[174] A prophesy of WW2?

relieved of the present darkness and led along the road to true light and life. As capacity for introspection develops a new Light begins to dawn and the way of life becomes clear. It is from introspection that all phenomena of the world take rise. It is through introspection alone that the human mind can attain unto light and see the true way.

Hitherto mankind has been looking in vain to religions like Christianity and Buddhism for the way of Light. These religions still dominate the mind of large sections of the human race. Man has now reached a stage, however, where such religions can do little to lead him toward his consummation. And Philosophy, Ethics and Science have failed no less signally than Religion to lead man toward his true goal, the kingdom of introspection, man's real kingdom of Heaven. The more man trusts to these vanities today the more hopelessly bewildered will he find himself and the darker will grow his hope. The present is indeed a time of real crisis for humanity. Unless we realize our mental paralysis and come to the true source of thought and life the future offers no light.

[175]Through a divine order I was born into this world to reveal the truth to mankind. In obedience to the divine call I am bound to transmit the truth entrusted to me to mankind everywhere. TAIREIDO is a divine message to the peoples of the earth. In the brief time that has elapsed since the truth was revealed to me and I began to practice TAIREIDO, so many persons of the highest character have been led to the truth and now rejoice in it as I do, that I cannot but desire the more earnestly to share it with all men. The disciples of TAIREIDO are found now in almost every section of East Asia. They come from all classes of human society. The truth of TAIREIDO has touched the heart of humanity everywhere it has been taught and practiced. To become acquainted with the principles of TAIREIDO is at once to yield to their supreme authority. As the truth of life dawns and the human mind begins to see the wonders of existence as never before, devotion to TAIREIDO is a matter of course. In my work of diffusing the great truth of TAIREIDO I find no argument necessary. A simple statement of the truth itself always proves sufficient. Bewilderment at once ceases, the mind perceives the light, introspection has its fruit and the individual attains unto perfect mental and physical soundness.

To the whole world, therefore, I call with insistent voice. To the multitudes lost to truth and life I appeal in their own interest to heed the message. Old

---

[175] These next two paragraphs are not in The Japan Magazine article in December 1918 towards the end of this book, even though the paragraphs before and after these two paragraphs are included.

things are passing away and behold all things now are becoming new. Each must see that he has his place and part in the new age. What is worn out should be cast away and the new accepted the new thought that is the essence of life, the secret of true existence. O that all may be ready to receive the Light and Grace that transcend all earthly things, that both mind and body may be renewed according to truth and eternal life.

An Appeal to the World

One of the most impressive facts of the last hundred years has been the marvellous progress of physical science. So rapid and far-reaching has been the increase of knowledge and invention that if our ancestors should return to the earth they would faint with sheer amazement. A century ago not even the most sanguine of prophets would have dared to predict such progress as modern civilization has attained. Yet no one who has closely observed the real condition of human life will deny that its improvement has not kept pace with its material prosperity. Indeed it is open to grave doubt whether, side by side with this material advancement, man has shown any adequate sign of development or evolution. How far humanity has evolved during the past century may be inferred from the recent warlike state of Europe. While our ancestors would doubtless be astonished at the outward progress of their posterity, they would undoubtedly be correspondingly shocked at their lack of mental and moral development.

The civilization of our time is essentially nothing more than the materialization and mechanization of humanity. As the scientist resolves all substances into atoms, so any accurate analysis of mankind today reveals only a mass of mediocrity, as the atoms of matter, mere automata without a mind to master the body that clothes them. What better than a machine is the average person we know! Humanity seems to have lost all consciousness of its inherent greatness; man no longer exhibits the enduring and substantial character of his ancestors. There are of course, some indications of humanity awakening to a sense of what has been lost; there are signs of a desire to recover man's natural greatness and to escape from the coils of our soulless and mechanical civilization. But there is very little progress in the realization of man's dawning desire.

[176]Eucken and Bergson and Tagore have been lecturing mankind on want of deeper interest in mental and spiritual advancement, but they have added to the sum of human thought nothing that has not been found in the teachings

[176] This paragraph is not included in The Japanese Magazine article of 1918 at the end of this book.

of Buddha and Christ. Certainly our modern teachers have given us nothing more worthy of veneration than the teachers of the past. Unless our capacity for introspection surpasses that of these teachers there is a dark outlook indeed for humanity. If the present system of thought is persisted in we are destined to the denationalization of the Indians and Jews.

While amply aware of the progress of our material civilization we do not honestly desire to be enmeshed in its coils or ground in its machinery; and while recognizing the degree of thought achieved by our ancestors we cannot but admit its great distance from absolute perfection and truth. What man most wants is a spiritual civilization transcending the present material civilization as far as the latter now transcends the former. The thought of today, on which man's real progress depends, should transcend the civilization of today and the thought of the past. Only as man approaches this spiritual civilization will he attain unto the mind and culture of the real superman, that divine state which transcends all mind and matter.

No study of the past or present, however profound, can bring any peace or satisfaction to the soul of man, no matter how much he may value them. While material advancement goes on, mental and spiritual progress lags behind, and man is unable to face the new duties that constantly arise. Into this gulf between matter and mind, material civilization and mental progress, comes the new revelation to man, known as TAIREIDO, the essential essence of all things created and uncreated, the only reality that transcends matter and mind, and yet the foundation of all mental and material development. TAIREIDO is not the product but the producer of thought. Because of its absence from the materialistic civilization of today the world is threatened with human retrogression.

The Art of Reishi, which is the system by which TAIREIDO manifests its power in human life, imparts to man the divine capacity to reach his full consummation of mind and body. Thereby man attains to spiritual supremacy over matter, especially the substance of which he is composed. Man is more than the bodily raiment that encloses his spirit. TAIREIDO enables man to transcend mind and matter, to rise above the confusions of philosophy, science and religion.

Having devoted my life to this truth I can vouch for its reality, as can the thousands who have tested it and found it true. Therefore with the most absolute assurance I proclaim to the world the doctrine of TAIREIDO, knowing that only through acquirement of this truth can mankind attain unto transcendent thought, and the transcendent life that is its certain fruit.

[177]In this way come the new man and the divine civilization. My one hope is that the people of the world will respond to my earnest appeal and come into this body of transcendent thought and life, thus realizing their divine destiny and contribute toward the salvation of the world. Then the truly perfect world comes, for which all mankind is travailing in pain together until now.

Principles of Reiri-Gaku[178]

1. Reiri-Gaku and Science

TAIREIDO is the law of thought or essence of life on which all existence, human and divine, is based. Without it there can be no true thought and consequently no true development of human society. It is a system of thought; and it involves principles which are unchanging. The study of these divine and eternal principles is known as Reiri-Gaku, which covers the entire subject both theoretically and practically, dealing with the origin and action of transcendent phenomena as revealed in the past and present. Hitherto the phenomena of the material world have been relegated to the realm of physics, and the phenomena of the world that transcends the physical and psychological. Operations of the Divine have been left to the mental vagaries of the spiritualist or to the puerile skepticism of the materialist, which denies the existence of the Divine for lack of adequate thought. But any close and honest observation of the universe reveals action transcending man's mental and material experience. Reiri-Gaku takes one through a careful study of the principles of divine transcendence, as revealed in nature and mind.

2. Reiri-Gaku and Science

Modern civilization regards Science as the pivot on which all progress turns. All theory and practice must submit to scientific scrutiny and be thus approved before legitimate application is admitted. Yet in regard to the First Cause and its relation to mind and matter Science has no adequate answer, no reasonable explanation, not even a suggestion as how man may utilize the transcendent and divine. No progress in this direction can be made by depending on Science. This is admitted by all contemporary scholarship. And the reason is clear: all contemporary science is based on materialism. It knows nothing apart from physical phenomena. The cause and actual

---

[177] Unlike the preceding paragraphs, this paragraph is not part of The Japanese Magazine article of 1918 at the end of this book.

[178] Reiri-Gaku = the study of TAIREIDO

substance or reality of phenomena science tells nothing about. Psychology has its own system of metaphysics, but they do not adequately deal with the cause and import of mental and spiritual phenomena. Consequently the system of thought on which modern civilization is based wanders along a bifurcated path of materialism and spiritualism that leads to vexed conclusions or else to nowhere!

Reiri-Gaku deals with the system of TAIREIDO, or new thought, the way of the eternal substance and essence of things, recognizing the two elements of matter and spirit, and showing the one element of Reishi as their origin and maintenance. Reishi being the essential cause of all things, matter and spirit are its consequent phenomena. Reishi, or Spirit-action, has its origin in TAIREI, or Supreme Spirit, the underlying essence of all existence. Taireido reveals and explains the fundamental principles of Tairei; and as Tairei is absolute TRUTH, transcending all time and space, existence and non-existence, knowledge of its principles lifts the mind of man to a plane of transcendence over mind and matter. Being the supreme and transcendent light it leads man along the path of Truth, and imparts to him the thought and power essential to the consummation of human life. In other words, man acquires the Art of Reishi, the power to act as the Author of all true action does. Reishi involves cause and effect, origin and creation, motion and transformation, the power of inorganic mutation and the spirit of organic life. In Reiri-Gaku, TAIREI, the fundamental substance, produces one element Reishi; and the one element of Reishi is the cause of the two elements known as matter and spirit. To TAIREIDO, therefore, there is no contradiction between matter and spirit, both of which are the results of Reishi.

Reiri-Gaku does not disapprove of the principles of modern physical and metaphysical science so far as they follow the path of truth as indicated by Taireido. The great imperfection of modern Science as a guide to Truth must be admitted, as its chief attention is devoted to phenomena and their consequences, leaving such fundamental questions as primary cause out of count altogether. For the proper study of these essential questions of our existence Reiri-Gaku is the only perfect science known to man. It comprehends fully the truths of all physical and metaphysical science, as well as the great fundamental truths transcending the sphere of mind and matter. And so in the system of Reiri-Gaku, all the facts of modern science are given due place and consideration.

3. Life's Interpretation

Speaking broadly, the universe may be regarded as phenomena of life. Every human being is conscious of the possession of life. Physical science considers human life as composition of certain materials, and metaphysics takes human life as manifestation of spirit. Material science affirms that life is the result of a chemical combination of sixteen elements, and asserts that what we call life is no more than an exhibition of these elements in combined action. The metaphysicians, on the other hand, hold that life is a manifestation of spiritual power, that matter is inert without some spiritual or metaphysical force to give it motion. Life can only come from life. Spontaneous generation is not proven. Once life departs from the body death supervenes, and the same material that once lived, lives no more. Life has departed because it is a thing apart from and above matter. It has, therefore, a separate existence. According to the teaching of Reiri-Gaku neither of these contentions has regard to absolute truth. It is futile to speak of the action of spirit apart from matter, or of the action of matter apart from spirit. It is only as body and spirit are combined that life can be recognised. A materialistic conception of life is as false as a purely spiritual conception of it. No conception is legitimate or true that does not involve both mind and matter.

Now Reiri-Gaku recognizes the truth of existence as it is, and not as modern science would have it to be; the material and spiritual are considered as united and one, and the spiritual is looked upon as supreme over the material, both being the products of Reishi, the secret of all life. There can be no manifestation of life without Reishi: life is Reishi in action. Reishi, the essence of Life, produces inorganic matter as well as organic life. Both body and spirit are, therefore, the product of Reishi and the manifestation of life. Matter and life are phenomena of Reishi in action. It is, therefore, but natural that those who study the phenomena of the Universe from a purely material point of view, as well as those who study life from a purely spiritual point of view, should both be equally in error and fail to reach the truth of things. Those who desire to become one with the truth of things as they are, and realize the cause as well as the consequence of the substance of life, must take up the study of Reiri-Gaku.

4. The Supreme Aim

Reiri-Gaku imparts to man the supreme aim of existence. It takes the mind through a theoretical examination of the essential substance of matter and mind and the power underlying them. The student thus acquires a perfect knowledge of the action and the application of Reishi by which true development of mind and body can be attained, a perfect human being produced, and the supreme happiness and peace of the individual achieved. Reiri-Gaku thus does for mankind what no other system of science or thought has ever even pretended to do.

The Internal Action of Reishi

1. Mental and Physical Training Necessary to Acquirement of the Art

The Internal Action of Reishi can be acquired only after having acquired the Art of External Action of Reishi, and not before. Having once acquired mastery of the External Action, mastery of the Internal Action of Reishi is easy. Mastery of the Internal Action of Reishi, however, is not quite as simple as is the acquirement of the art of applying the External Action. The progress made depends a good deal on whether one has the privilege of being under a master of the Art or has to depend on book directions. After long study and patient elaboration of tested methods we have prepared plans enabling anyone to acquire the Art of the Internal Action of Reishi from studying a following the directions laid down in this volume.

It is our duty to impress on the student the sacredness of the book, which is the outcome of revelations of truth to the author in his long search for light on the meaning of life. He offers it to mankind as a precious gift, bearing light on the divine world, so that by following the light, mankind may become acquainted with the secret of existence and knows how to live. To make progress in the prudent and sincere, carefully perusing the book and observing its directions, so that success may be assured.

In order to acquire the Art of the Internal Action of Reishi preparation of mind and body is not different from that required for the acquirement of the Art of the External Action of Reishi. The point of supreme importance is to see that one acquires the Art of making External Action of Reishi become an Internal Action as well. When the Internal Action is transmitted from one organic or inorganic substance to another, the transmission produces the External Action of Reishi. When one who is under the influence of the External Action of Reishi presses the Reishi Board, for example, it moves; but that does not mean that the action of Reishi is transmitted to the board. The board naturally moves when subjected to the transmission of the Action of Reishi, but it does not possess the Action as the transmitter does. The board, therefore, does not move of itself, but under the power of the Action of Reishi. It moves only when the whole of the board is under the influence of the Action of Reishi.

In such manner one is subjected to the Action of Reishi by the practitioner of the Art. He is in the same condition of mind as when under the External Action of Reishi, that is, in a state of mental transcendence, a condition transcending his usual self, to attain which his mind must be in a proper condition, for any unnatural state of mind obstructs the Internal Action of Reishi. The Action of Reishi is not produced by putting forth physical strength or by pressing the Reishi board. The board is first very lightly touched by the palm, leaving it to move itself. As the Internal Action of Reishi can be transmitted by a good practitioner in any direction to anyone or anything, it sometimes passes through the board into the floor, in which case the board does not move, for it is not possible for both the board and the floor to move under such influence. In case the Action passes through the board into the floor, the board is given motion by the other hand, when it will move instantly. If the other hand fails to give the board this assistance and it only left to itself, the divine movement may not appear, as the Action is transmitted wholly through the board into what is underneath. This is a very important fact to bear in mind.

2. The Reishi Board[179]

In acquiring the Art of the Internal Action of Reishi the instrument known as the Reishi Board is indispensable. The board is made of *hinoki* wood, and is about 7 inches long and 4 wide and an inch thick. It should be planed as smooth as possible. The board must be a semicircle in shape, its angles facial. The board may be varnished or lacquered on both sides, but it is better without such coating. The wood must be completely seasoned and dry.

The beginner uses only a single board, but the number is increased gradually with the progress of the practitioner to 20, 30, 50 and even 100 boards, according to the progress made in the Art. The student should have the boards prepared beforehand, so as to have them ready as wanted. Trays, books, or other such flat articles, may be used instead of boards, but the cumulative effect of the Internal Action of Reishi and its transmission are best experienced when using boards. It must be borne in mind that the board is necessary only while one is training in the Art. One thorough practiced in the Internal Action of Reishi has no further use for the board. When

[179] These experiments in Internal Transmission of Reishi would be very interesting to see in relation to the transmission of Reiki.

applying the Art of Reishi to the removal of disease no board is necessary. One who has progressed so little in the Art as to find the board still a necessity would not be able to affect a cure.

The board may be made of any other wood besides that named, if one likes. The wood of the paulownias tree is best for beginners. Even before one has advanced very far in the Art he can move as many as 100 pieces of this wood, one on the other. The coarser the quicker the transmission of the Action. But even the finest of wood can transmit the Action, though more slowly than wood of a coarser grain. And the same applies to mineral substance. Flat pieces of mineral may be made into boards for the practice of the Internal Action of Reishi. In all cases, as before intimated, a board is necessary for the acquirement of the Art of Internal Action of Reishi. After one has made sufficient progress with the boards, he may try his Art on desks, tables, chairs or anything he fancies. Inevitable success indicates great advancement in the Art.

3. How to Make Progress

Lay the palm of the hand flat on the Reishi Board, with fingers together, and press so as to produce the Internal Action of Reishi. The method can be taught successfully either by verbal or personal instruction, but not so easily by book instruction. If when one presses the board, the External Action of Reishi alone is produced it is useless. The hand must be brought close to the board without inducing the External Action and then wait until the board moves itself. The beginner must remember that it will take him some little time to succeed in transmitting the Internal Action of Reishi to the board.

The time may vary from a few seconds to a few minutes, for one who is learning, to produce freely and at will the Internal Action of Reishi. See the photograph illustrating the action here described.

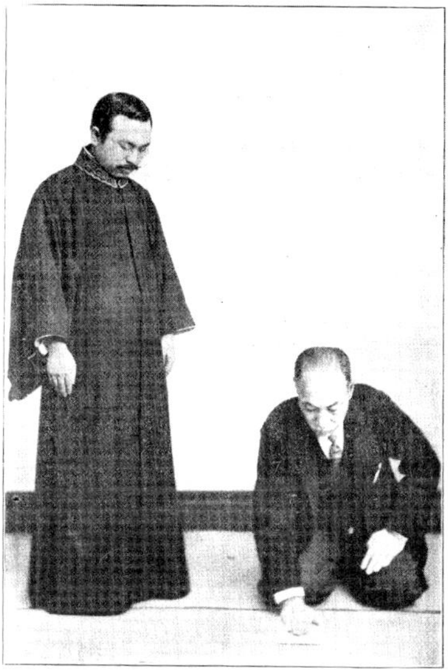

MOVING REISHI BOARD
By Assistant Kawaguchi

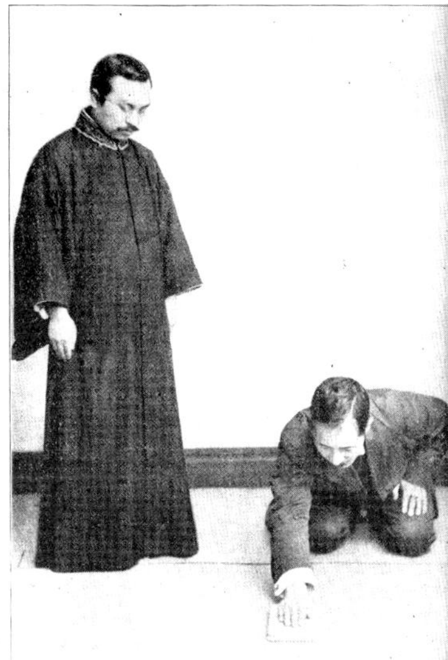

MOVING TWO BOARDS BY REISHI ACTION
By Assistant Hasegawa

The beginner should exercise the method very calmly and deliberately, as at first he may have difficulty in distinguishing between the Internal and the External Action of Reishi, the latter being produced at times instead of the former. When but one Reishi board is employed, it often revolves violently, but with two the Action is not so violent, the movement being rather more moderate. Should the practitioner in his eagerness try to cause two boards to move as violently as one, the two boards will slip past each other and fail to transmit the action. The state of mind necessary to the transmission of the Internal Action of Reishi is just the same in the case of two boards as when practicing with one. See the illustration referring to the use of two boards.

The next step after mastering two boards is to try three. These in turn will prove slow in receiving the influence of the Action than two boards. Haste is fatal here. One must wait patiently and calmly for the manifestation of the Internal Action of Reishi, until the Action is transmitted to all three and they begin to move of themselves. The External Action of Reishi is especially liable to arise in this case, and care must be taken to avoid inducing it. When the three boards, under the Internal Action of Reishi, go forward of themselves, the practitioner may congratulate himself that he has made great progress in the Art. Indeed he may then conclude that he has passed his first examination. But the beginner should repeat the Action with one, two and three boards, many times, so as to assure himself that he has mastered it. See the illustration concerning the use of three boards.

Having successfully transmitted the Internal Action of Reishi to three boards the student may then try his Art on five, but he may take four if he likes. But it is easier to transmit the Action to five boards, if the practitioner has already mastered the Art of moving three. Lay the five boards carefully on each other in a pile. They must lie close or the Action will not be transmitted. To succeed in moving five boards is a critical stage, and the student should proceed with great care and perseverance; for if he now succeeds he will have little difficulty thereafter. Note the accompanying illustration.

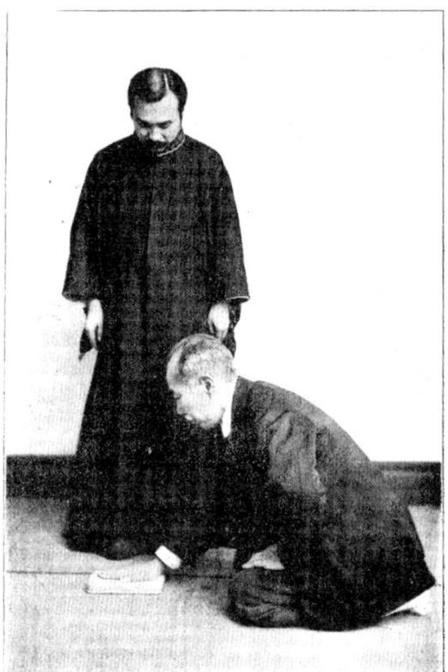

MOVING THREE BOARDS
By Assistant Kawaguchi

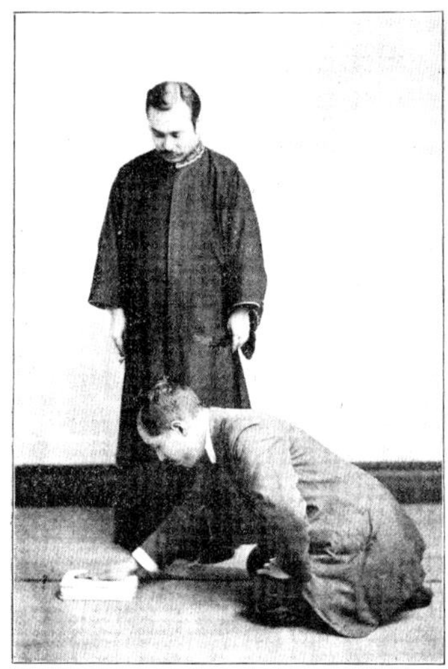

MOVING FIVE BOARDS
By Assistant Hasegawa

The successful student may now pass on to practicing on ten boards at once, for it is easy to transmit the Internal Action of Reishi to ten boards as to five, once you know how. The boards will move and go forward of themselves in the same manner as did the five boards, unless there be some obstructing medium. There must be no attempt to move them. Let boards move themselves. It usually takes about two whole days of practice before the learner can succeed in transmitting the Internal Action of Reishi to ten boards, although some have succeeded in one day, and others have taken a number of days. See illustration.

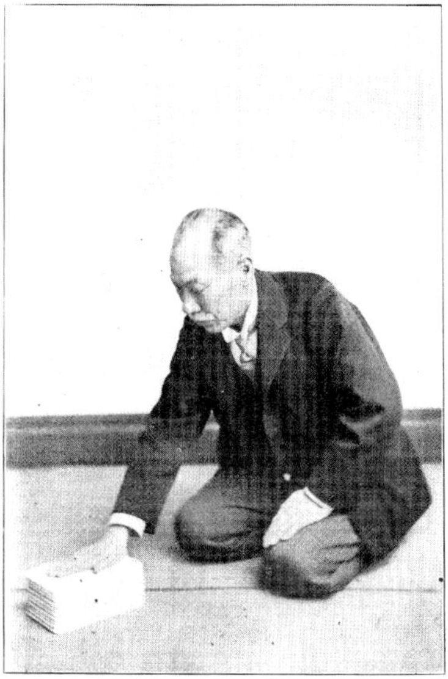

TEN BOARDS MOVED BY REISHI
By Assistant Kawaguchi

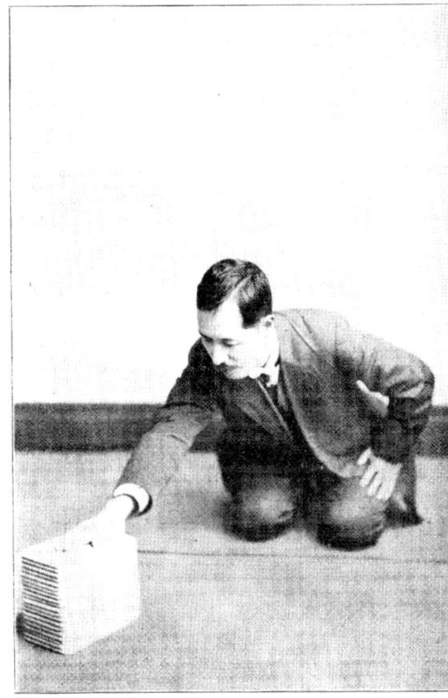

TWENTY BOARDS MOVING BY REISHI
By Assistant Hasegawa

After succeeding in transmitting the Internal Action of Reishi to ten boards, as many as twenty may be tried next. It takes no more art to move twenty than ten if one knows how. One may proceed from 13, 15, and 17 up to 20 if one so desires. But one makes more rapid progress in the Art by rising to twenty instead of working up gradually to that number.

From successful use of twenty one may proceed to try thirty. This is an interesting experiment; for when the practitioner can effectively transmit the Internal Action of Reishi to thirty boards he has qualified for the healing of disease. This is the testing point of his capacity to cure. He must therefore assure himself that he has really succeeded in transmitting the Internal Action of Reishi to thirty boards. If one is not perfect in mastering the art in regard to thirty, it is no use for him to go higher, for he would not be successful with more. Consequently when one has succeeded in moving thirty boards the practice should be repeated often for the sake of assurance and confidence. It is essential to perfection of the Art that the boards should move of themselves, and not by the help of anything mental or physical, which must be avoided as far as possible.

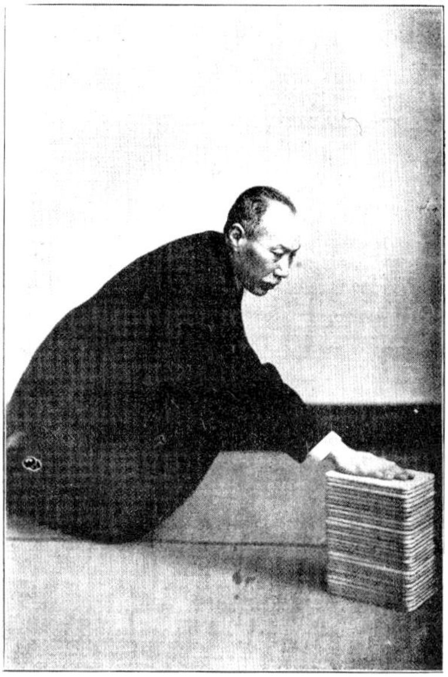

SUCCESSFUL MOVEMENT OF THIRTY BOARDS
By Assistant Kawaguchi

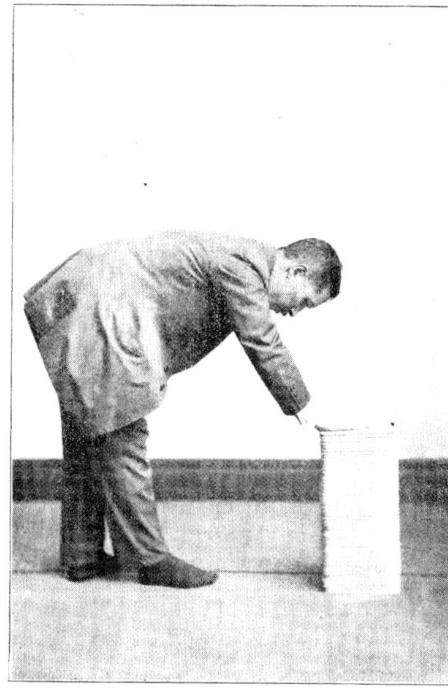

FIFTY BOADS SUCCESSFULLY MOVED BY REISHI
By Assistant Hasegawa

After successfully passing the critical test of thirty boards the student may now go up to the use of fifty, either at once or gradually, as he feels inclined. To succeed in moving fifty boars is to have acquired a fine mastery of the Art. It is impossible to practice the Art of moving from thirty to fifty Reishi boards while sitting: one must invariably stand. At first it may seem to the practitioner a hopeless endeavor to transmit the Internal Action of Reishi to as many as fifty boards, but a diligent exercise of the Art will succeed in so doing.

One who can effectively transmit the Internal Action of Reishi to fifty boards may consider himself perfectly qualified to cure almost any kind of disease or bodily ailment. But to acquire a still greater portion of the divine power he must add twenty-five. It is distinctly more boards to his list to try his power on seventy-five. It is distinctly more difficult to move this number than to move fifty. But when the action is effectively transmitted, it will go through the boards and move all of them; and when that vital moment arrives when he sees the boards all move forward he feels a pleasure of triumph beyond all words. There is no disease that will not disappear before such a master of the Art of Reishi.

The maximum number of boards that can be moved by the Internal Action of Reishi is one hundred. More may be tried, but one hundred are enough for all purposes of the Art, which is simply to secure sufficient power to heal disease and regulate the body to a perfect state. The difference between one's mastery of one board as a beginner and one's mastery of one hundred boards as a master of the Art of the Internal Action of Reishi is vast indeed, as no one knows better than the master himself. He now feels that he can transmit the Action of Reishi through anything. Though the method ends with pressing the palm on one hundred boards and causing them to move by the Internal Action of Reishi, yet the Art does not end there: it is infinite. There are other methods to be taken up if one is to go on and learn.

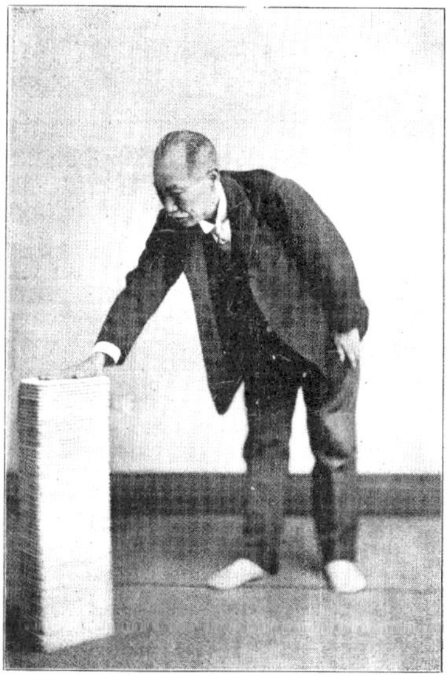

MOVING SEVENTY-FIVE BOARDS
By Assistant Kawaguchi

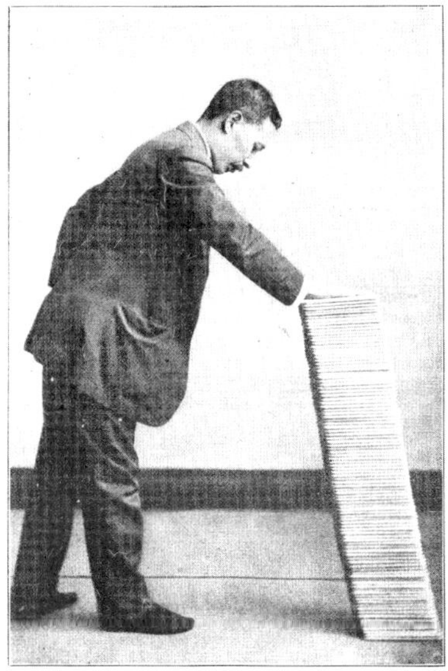

MOVING ONE HUNDRED BOARDS
By Assistant Hasegawa

4. Rotatory Internal Action of Reishi

The Rotatory Internal Action of Reishi begins with taking one Reishi board and pressing it with the palm of the hand, the fingers being close together, after the manner of the palm-pressing process. When the Internal Action is successfully transmitted the board moves gently forward. The practitioner should follow it up as lightly as possible. Soon the board increases speed until it runs around the room. If the practitioner closes his eyes the Internal Action of Reishi will be more quickly transmitted; but as soon as the board moves forward the eyes must be opened. See illustration.

When the Reishi board attains rapid speed the practitioner should still follow it as lightly as possible, keeping the palm pressed closely to the board. Then the board will attain a very rapid speed, as if pulling the hand with it, until finally it circles around the room so fast that the practitioner has difficulty in keeping up with it. Finally the speed attained is so rapid as to be beyond that of the practitioner and he falls exhausted, while the board continues to speed around the room[180]. See illustration.

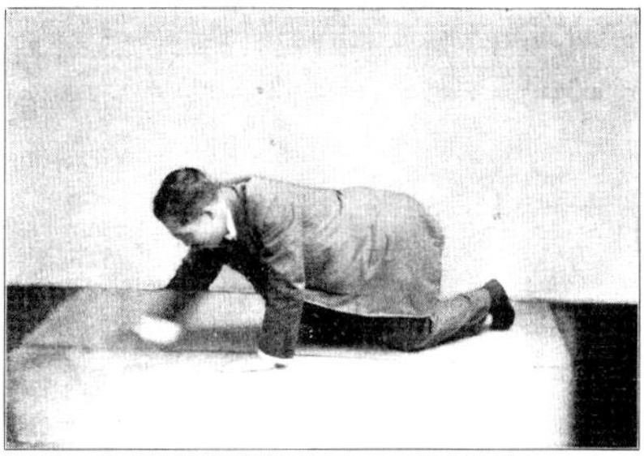

REISHI BOARD ATTAINS GREAT SPEED
By Assistant Kawaguchi

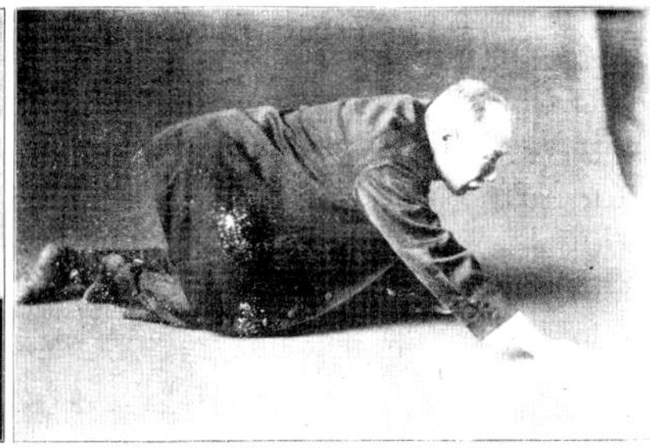

BOARD MOVED BY ROTATORY, NTIERNAL ACTION OF REISHI
By Assistant Kawaguchi

When the board attains a speed of such violence as to appear to draw the hand of the practitioner after it, he should cease to exert any pressure and leave the board to its own movement, simply allowing his hand to be carried with it. The board then attains a rotatory motion beyond his control, flying off his hand. At the moment when the board attempts to leave the hand it should be pressed again so as not to lose touch with it; while at the same time care must be taken not to induce the External Action of Reishi, which retards the progress of the Art, though attention to this matter must not be such as to absorb the mind of the practitioner. See illustration.

---

[180] Care may be needed with such boards? Tanaka's descriptions suggest a similar effect to Ouija board, patented by Elijah Jefferson Bond on Feb 10th 1891. Or to when fingers placed lightly on a glass move it, sometimes fast.

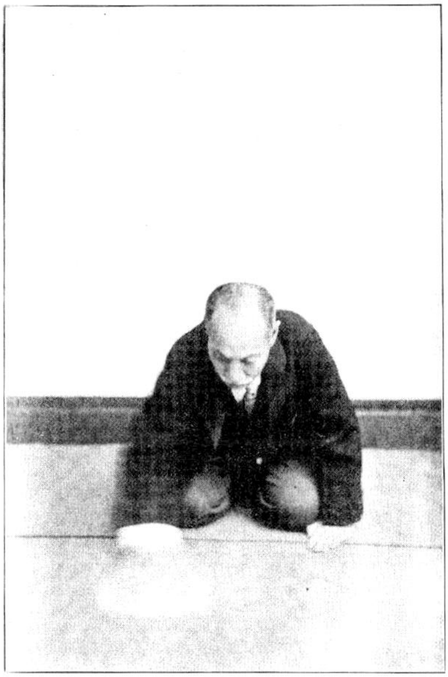

SUDDEN MOVEMENT OF BOARD BY HAND AND ONLY
By Assistant Kawaguchi

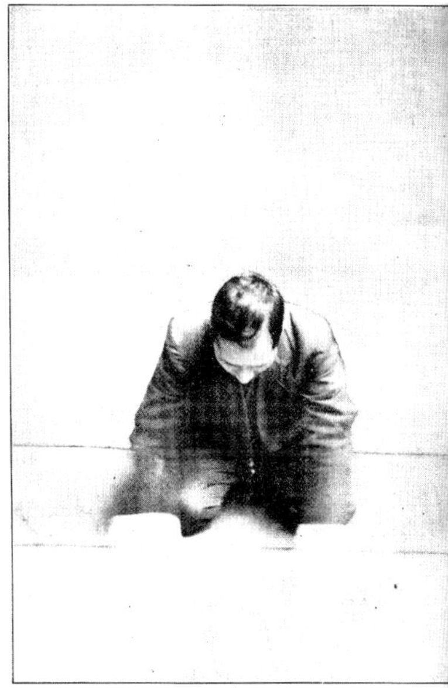

MOVING REISHI BOARD WITH BOTH HANDS
By Assistant Kawaguchi

As soon as the practitioner has succeeded in transmitting the Internal Action of Reishi to one board with the right palm, he should take a second board and transmit the Internal Action of Reishi to it with the left palm. The two boards will then rotate so violently that the practitioner feels as if they were floating on air. During this act care must be taken not to induce the External Action of Reishi, a thing very likely to occur at such a time; for the boards must rotate by force of Internal Action alone. The more successful the practitioner becomes in this practice of the Internal Action of Reishi, the more successful will he be in the curing of disease. The rotatory method must be confined to one board. that is, one to each hand, as in this process boards must not be piled on each other. See illustration.

5. Internal Skin Action of Reishi

This method consists in producing the Internal Action of Reishi in any portion of the skin. First the practitioner takes one board and tries to transmit to it the Internal Action of Reishi with the back of the hand, until it moves rapidly forward by itself. After thus succeeding with one hand, the number is increased; piling one on another until the Internal Action of Reishi is successfully transmitted to ten or twenty boards. Care should be taken not to press the boards too firmly. But sufficient strength must be exerted to keep the boards, thus piled up, close together. The practitioner should practice with both hands so as to be able to use either with equal facility.

When the practitioner succeeds in thus transmitting the Internal Action of Reishi through the skin of the back of the hand, he should try to do so through the skin of the arm. With proper practice and sufficient progress the student should be able easily to transmit the Internal Action in this way to from 20 to 50 boards. It is important to keep the body, especially the waist, as free as possible during practice, in order to have the boards move with as little obstruction as possible. The movement of the arm should meet with no hitch or interference of any kind. In the same way a successful practitioner can move the Reishi boards with the nose, the cheek, leg, finger tips, abdomen, back, or any part if the body that can be conveniently brought into contact with the board to transmit the Internal Action of Reishi thereto. The palm, the back of the hand and the arm are, however, the most convenient sections of contact for such practice.

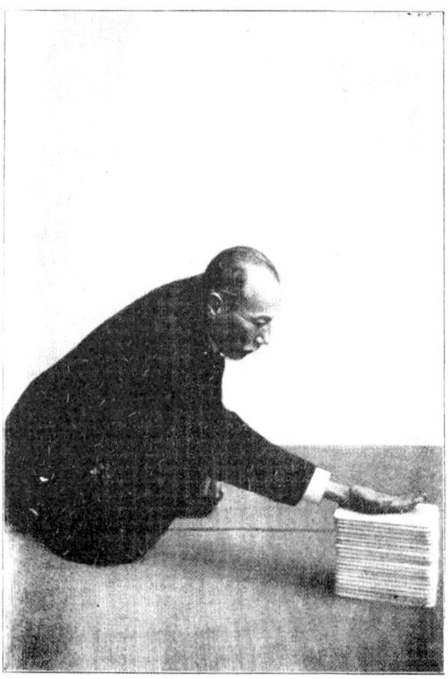

A TEST OF HAND SKIN REISHI POWER
By Assistant Kawaguchi

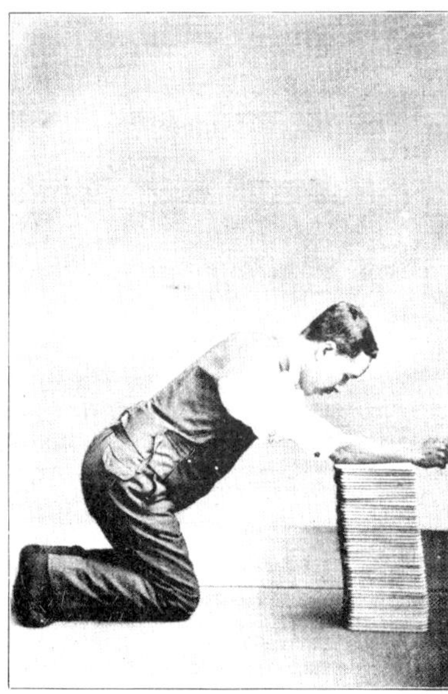

TEST OF ARM SKIN POWER
By Assistant Hasegawa

6. The Internal Nail Action of Reishi

The Internal Action of Reishi can be produced from even the nail ends, which means that it can readily be produced from any part of the body. The method consists in applying the four fingers without use of the thumb, touching the board with the ends of the nails, until it moves forward. The ends of the nails must be brought into contact with the board very slightly, with the fingers either close together or slightly apart. In this act care must be taken not to allow any part of the finger skin to touch the board. See illustration.

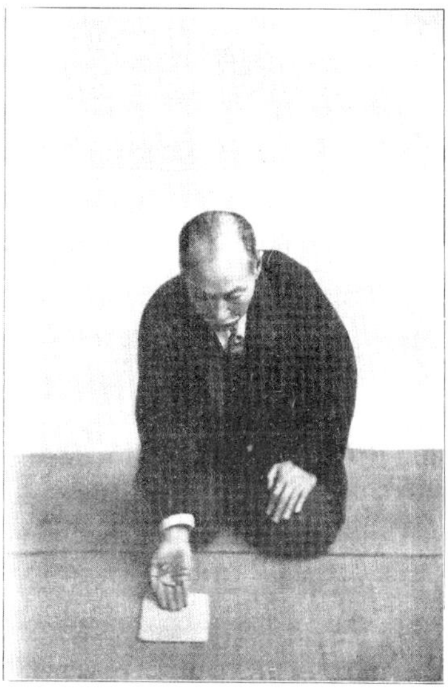

TESTING NAIL POWER
By Assistant Kawaguchi

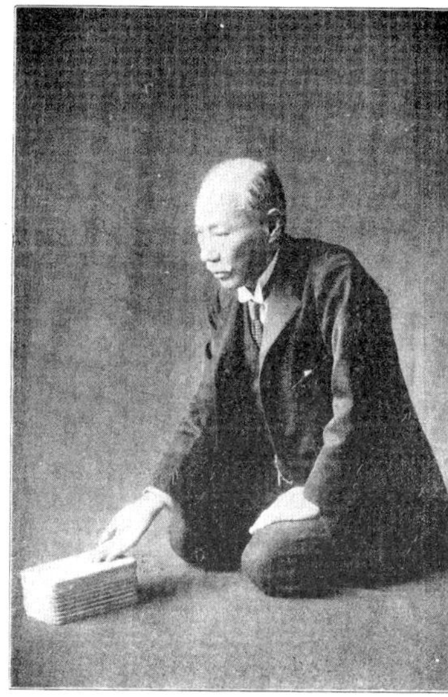

MOVING BOARD BY FINGER NAILS
By Assistant Kawaguchi

After assuring oneself of success with one board then two, three, four and five boards should be tried. One must not be disappointed if success does not attend every attempt at transmitting the Internal Action of Reishi in this way, especially if the practitioner be impatient or prone to undue haste. But he should not be satisfied until he has been able to increase the number of boards to at least five, although it is almost as easy to operate with ten boards. Upon attaining sufficient success with the nails, then the process should be attempted with the thumb only, after this with each of the remaining fingers.

7. Internal Action of Reishi by Conduction

The next step in the progress of acquiring capacity for the transmission of the Internal Action of Reishi is to place the Reishi boards end to end, one corner of the board just touching the corner of the other, the opposite angle being suspended by the right hand and the Internal Action of Reishi being transmitted from that angle. The Action passes from the board thus held obliquely to the one lying flat until both go forward at the same moment, the practitioner but lightly touching the board which he still holds obliquely as follows the other, so that it may not fall down. The practice should be carried out with each hand as well as with both hands simultaneously. See illustration.

Next the board should be laid flat and the other connected with it without being held obliquely, but vertically or horizontally, through the Internal Action of Reishi can be best transmitted when the board is held obliquely. When the boards are laid flat in succession, any number from two to ten may be used, while the number used as conductors of Internal Action of Reishi may be increased from two to five. The conducting board may be held vertically or placed horizontally on the one laying flat. One should gain facility in the use of either or both hands in this practice, especially as the number of boards increase. See illustration.

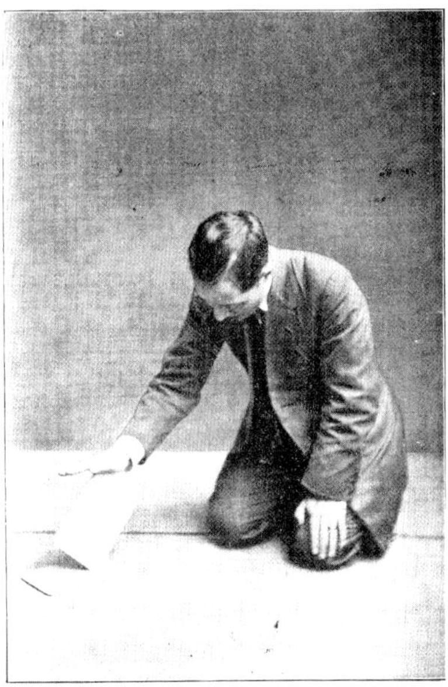

MOVING BOARD BY REISHI INDUCTION THROUGH ANOTHER BOARD
By Assistant Hasegawa

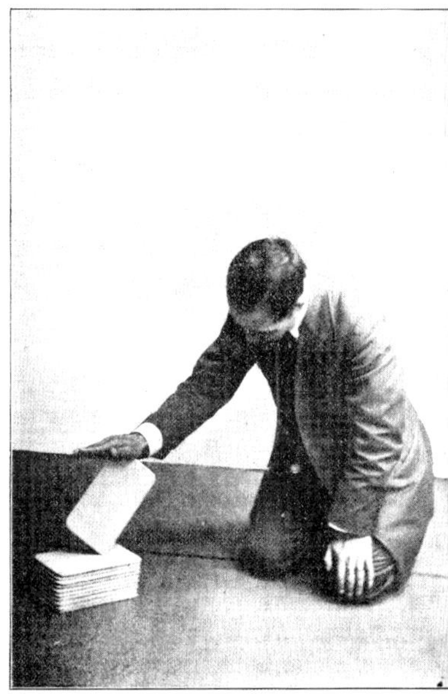

REISHI THROUGH A BOARD
By Assistant Hasegawa

8. Transmitting the Internal Action of Reishi to Tables

A table of either three or four legs may be used for this experiment. Lay the table upside down. Let two practitioners press the ends of the legs slightly with their palms, whereupon the Internal Action of Reishi will be transmitted to the whole table. As soon as the table thus receives the whole Action of Reishi it will begin to move slowly of itself in a rotatory motion. After a few revolutions the Action will be so rapid that the practitioners cannot follow it. The same phenomenon may be produced by even one practitioner if he places his palms on the ends of the legs. See illustration.

The next step in table Action is to place the table upright in the usual way, and transmit the Internal Action of Reishi to it with the palm in the regular manner, when the Action will be conveyed to the entire table, including even the legs, and it will then move of itself. The motion will become so rapid it will make it difficult for the practitioner to follow it. It is important to touch the table lightly at first and without any special occupation of mind on the part of the practitioner, leaving the table to move of itself. When beginning, the practitioner must close his eyes, and open them only after the movement has attained sufficient speed. See illustration.

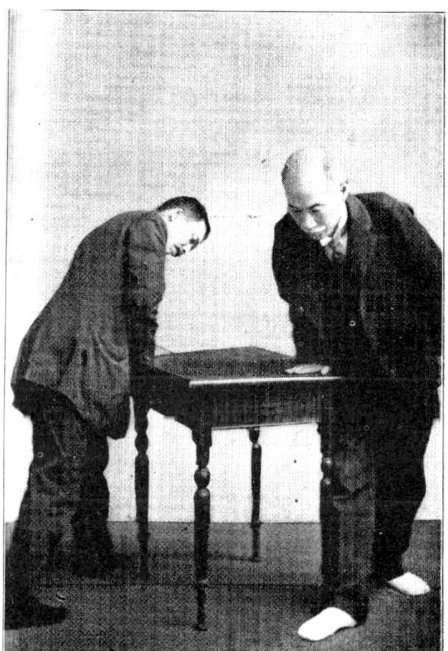

TRANSMITTING ACTION OF REISHI TO TABLE
By Assistants Kawaguchi and Hasegawa

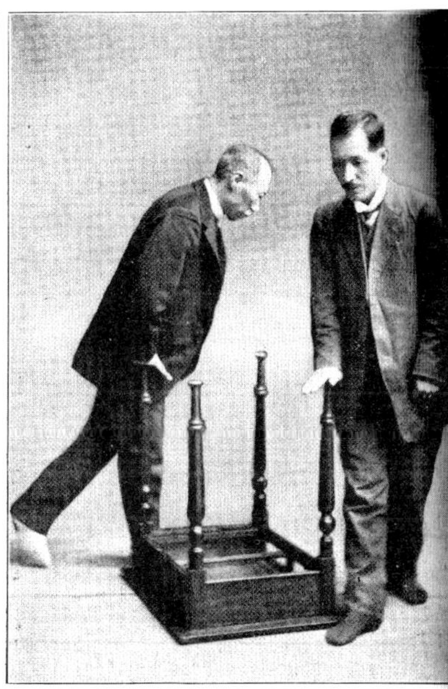

MOVING A TABLE BY REISHI
By Assistants Kawaguchi and Hasegawa

9. Transmission of the Internal Action to Chairs

The method varies according to the shape of the chair. The practitioner must seize some part of the chair firmly and transmit the Internal Action of Reishi to the chair. In a few minutes the Action will be transmitted to the whole chair, which begins at once to move of itself from the end of the legs until it goes forward. The practitioner must begin with closed eyes, and open them only when the chair begins to move forward rapidly, after which it may be left to pursue its own course, when it will move so fast that the practitioner cannot follow it even by running. The best way is to practice on two boards at first. Boards of from six to twelve feet in length and six inches wide are best, and of the same thickness as the usual Reishi board. The chair should be placed on these to begin with, when it will be found to move more quickly than if on some other surface. See illustration.

To make the chair move of itself the practitioner should take hold firmly of some part of the chair, and when he becomes able to transmit the Internal Action of Reishi he can do so by touching the chair lightly with the palm of the other hand as the centre of gravity, both palms being employed if necessary.

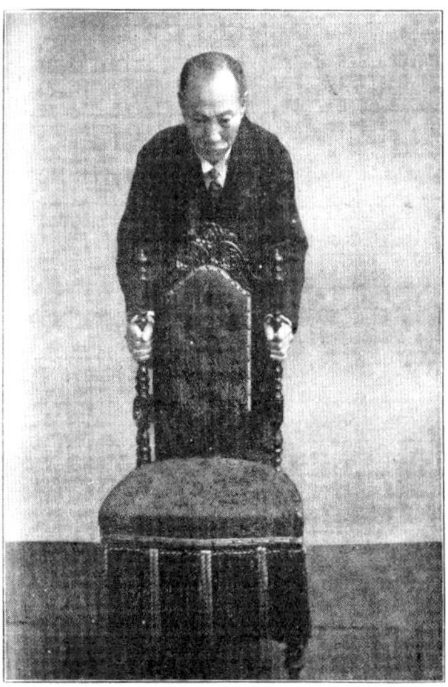

MOVING A CHAIR BY REISHI
By Assistant Kawaguchi

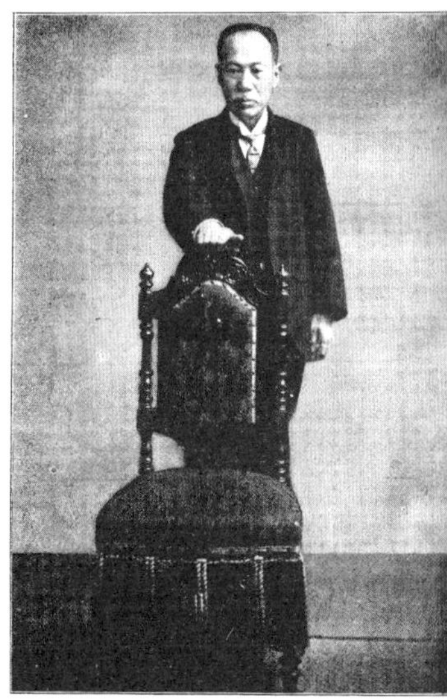

INTERNAL ACTION OF REISHI THROUGH A CHAIR
By Assistant Kawaguchi

Sometimes it may happen that the Internal Action is transmitted to the board on which the chair rests, when the chair presents a condition as if glued to the board and will not move. In such cases the practitioner should press one of the legs gently with the toe, just to start it. When the chair once begins to move it will attain a more rapid motion gradually and until finally it goes very fast. See Illustration.

Even a chair on which some one is seated will move of itself when given the Internal Action of Reishi. All the practitioner has to do is to seize some part of the chair convenient for transmission of the Internal Action, the one seated on the chair keeping his feet off the floor but in a natural posture. As soon as the whole chair receives the Internal Action of Reishi it begins to move slowly and with increasing speed. Care must be taken to keep the chair on the boards and not running beside them. The chair will move most lightly if two or more men act jointly in giving it the Internal Action of Reishi. See illustration.

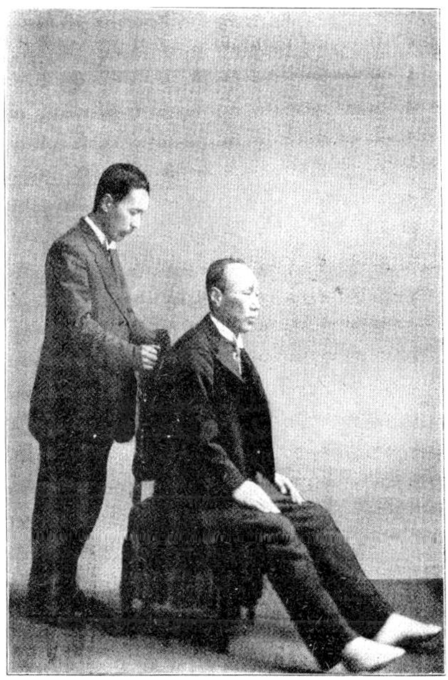

MOVING CHAIR WITH ONE SITTING ON IT
By Assistants Kawaguchi and Hasegawa

10. Transmitting the Internal Action of Reishi through Space

This wonderful Action is realized without any medium save two practitioners mutually co-operating at a distance. One of them sends the Action and the other receives it. First two practitioners may stand about two feet apart[181]. One of them closes the eyes and places the hands upon the knees, while the other imparts the Internal Action by inducing it through his right hand. That's when the hands of the receiver raise spontaneously and unconsciously. If the Action be transmitted to one hand only that hand rises; and if transmitted to two hands, both will rise. At such a moment it sometimes happens that the External Action of Reishi is induced violently in the receiver, which, if allowed to operate, will produce some very remarkable phenomena. See illustration.

It is to be borne in mind that the transmitter of the Internal Action must begin by bringing the muscles of his right hand to extreme tension, putting his full strength into the act, but after he becomes accustomed to the Act, this extreme tension is unnecessary. In most cases as soon as the practitioner raises his hand, with muscles tensed, the right hand of the receiver rises in response; and when the transmitter raises his left hand, the receiver will do the same.

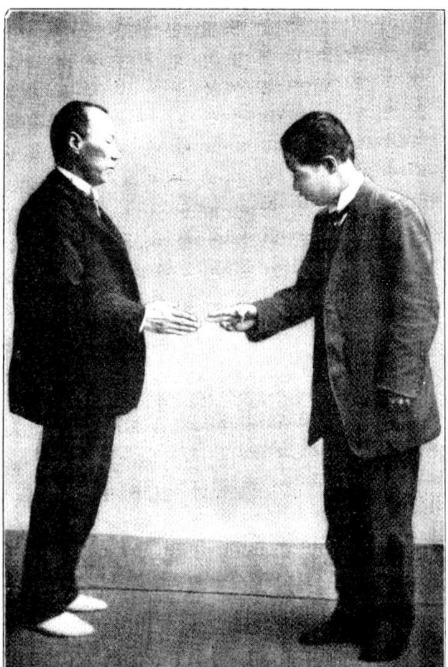

REISHI ACTION THROUGH SPACE
By Assistants Kawaguchi and Hasegawa

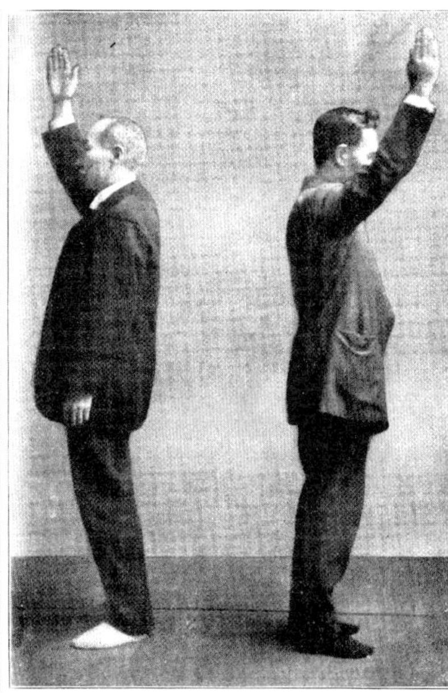

ANOTHER TRANSMISSION THROUGH SPACE
By Assistants Kawaguchi and Hasegawa

[181] Nowadays this action is often called, 'Beaming'

Sometimes it occurs that the receiver does not raise the same hand as the transmitter, when it must not supposed to be due to the intention of the transmitter, but simply to the fact that the Internal Action of Reishi had been imparted to the hand raised. Usually the raising of both hands by the transmitter causes the receiver likewise to raise both hands but it is not impossible that only one hand might be raised by the latter. When the receiver of the Internal Action raises both hands he sometimes falls backward under the influence. See illustration.

The transmission of the Internal Action of Reishi through space can be practiced either sitting or standing. Some receivers of the Internal Action of Reishi have the Action produced violently in their body, in which case it is necessary to check the Action somewhat. If the Action be no more violent than to cause the receiver to fall backward when he raises his hands, he may be allowed to do so. Such violence, however, is usually experienced only after considerable practice. As the practitioner becomes more and more successful the distance between them may be lengthened, until finally they can succeed in transmitting the Action over a space of sixty feet or so. See illustration.

When the transmitter and receiver stand face to face, the latter must close his eyes, though this is unnecessary, if they stand back to back. It is better at first for the two to stand from two to six feet apart. The transmitter raises his right hand in the manner directed above, when the receiver will also raise his right hand; and as soon as the transmitter raises his left hand the receiver also raises his left hand. This is the normal Action whether the distance is two feet or sixty feet. It is in this way that one proves that the Action of Reishi transcends consciousness and distance.

Hints on Acquiring the Internal Action of Reishi

After the practitioner of Reishi has fully acquired the processes described in the preceding paragraphs, and is able by the pressure of the palm to transmit the Internal Action of Reishi to boards, tables, chairs and to others, as well as by using the back of the hand or the nails, and can also transmit the Internal Action of Reishi through space, he can begin to feel that he has made good progress and is a capable practitioner. It must be remembered, as has been indicated more than once in these pages, that to convey the whole truth of the matter concerning Reishi is very difficult to do in writing, as some of the forms and processes are not easy to describe in words, though it would be very easy to illustrate them in personal instruction. But the student may be assured that the methods above outlined are quite effective in producing the Action of Reishi. If success be not forthcoming it can only be through some misunderstanding of the directions given.

It is most important to understand the method of using palm pressure as the fundamental condition of transmitting the Internal Action of Reishi. A proper acquirement of this part of the Art is vital to success. Consequently the practitioner must drill himself assiduously in the processes described in the preceding pages from numbers 1 to 10. Assured of his ability to transmit the Internal Action of Reishi through on hundred boards the practitioner may have no doubt of his ability to cure all disease. The rotatory methods later adopted are for the purpose of giving further assurance of increased capacity, and to show how remarkable is the capacity possessed by the practitioner, but all is the result of developing the methods outlined in the earlier experiments. The beginning of the capacity depends on correct action in the pressure of the palm, in which one must take the keenest interest so as to start aright and acquire the fundamental principles of the Art. It has already been pointed out that books or pieces of pasteboard may be used as objects if boards are not at hand or convenient. Some students find that they are more successful by using other methods besides, or instead of, the pressure of the palm. The student must use the method he finds most successful. It is well to try all methods, but to make sure one is expert and well practiced in one method. Efficiency should be sought first in the method one finds easiest; and then go on to the other methods afterwards.

Many of the other methods are such as cannot be explained well in writing and therefore have been omitted from this book[182]. But the methods outlined above are sufficient if the student is earnest, intelligent and persevering; and once successful there is no further difficulty in treating disease. As the principal purpose of this book is to assist in preparing the practitioner for the treatment of disease, irrelevant methods are not discussed here. After one has proved himself capable of transmitting the Internal Action of Reishi by the methods suggested in this book, it will be time enough for him to turn his attention to other methods[183]. If keen and persistent he may be able to devise other methods himself, which will enable him to understand how very mysterious and wonderful the Internal Action of Reishi is.

---

[182] Suggesting that Tanaka taught additional information on his courses

[183] Again suggesting Tanaka taught students extra methods

He will find that the Internal Action of Reishi can be transmitted to plants and minerals with the same mysterious results as when transmitted to the objects suggested in the directions for practice given in this book. As regards the transmission of the Internal Action of Reishi there is no need to think of the conductor of this mysterious power. But of course when the Internal Action of Reishi is transmitted to animals and living things the results are always more wonderful than when transmitted to inanimate objects. Transmission to any hard or coarse substance is comparatively easy; but transmission successfully to the more delicate and refined organism of living tissue is much more difficult. It must, therefore, be understood at the start that inorganic substance always receives the Internal Action of Reishi more readily than organic substance. But this does not alter the fact that there is no substance impervious to the Internal Action of Reishi. There are only differences of susceptibility, involving greater practice and training in the Art, if the practitioner is to be successful. If it be more difficult to transmit the Internal Action of Reishi to organic substances than to inorganic by the usual mode of contact, it is still more difficult to transmit the Action without contact and at a distance. But in any case the palm pressure method will always prove the most effectual. In one way it is found that the organic substance, however, usually receives the Internal Action of Reishi better at a distance than in close proximity.[184]

When the student has mastered the methods directed in this book and completely proves capable of transmitting the Internal Action of Reishi, he can transmit the Internal Action of Reishi to anything, whether organic or inorganic. It cannot be said that transmission of the Internal Action of Reishi is absolutely independent of psychic action or physiological conditions, as it must always be transmitted by a living body. It is only from a human being that the Action of Reishi comes. But the Action of Reishi is not produced by psychical or physiological conditions, or by any combined action of these, but it is produced by the Source of life and power and may be transmitted by the person in whom it is produced to other persons or substances. When the Internal Action of Reishi is simply transmitted to inorganic substance there may be no great value or significance in the action, save as proving the capacity of the practitioner. But when the Action is transmitted to a living body the result is very significant and valuable, as is shown by resultant phenomena. It proves that the practitioner has the power to heal disease, which is one of the main purposes of transmitting the Internal Action of Reishi. How beneficial this Art is and must be, in the face so much failure

[184] Interesting to note and to see how Reiki practitioners have faired in these aspects of the Art.

on the part of medicine and doctors must be apparent to everyone. The use of the Art of the Internal Action of Reishi proves that what was once supposed to be incurable is not really so: all affection of the mind and body may be removed and normal conditions restored by the Art of Reishi, the power which originates all life, and regulates it. Modern medicine, as has been already said in these pages, is based on materialism, whereas life is not so based. TAIREIDO recognizes that life and spirit are supreme over all material and substance. The healing of disease must, therefore, be a spiritual action! It is a cooperation of soul, life and body to res the proper action and function of Reishi in the body and mind. Thus Reishi is an Art far beyond anything possible to medical science as we know it today[185]. Doubtless medical science will some time come to a development where it will rise above its present materialistic basis and reach the ideal of TAIREIDO; but then it will have ceased to be medicine. It will then have come to be a spiritual and divine art instead of a purely materialistic experiment that more often fails than succeeds.

Why should intelligent people await improvement in medicine while the divine Art of Reishi is now available and able to res all defects in the human mind and body? Medical science has been studying the needs of the human body for centuries; and if it were able to meet the demands of the body they would have been met long ago. Man is but a small thing after all, a mere insect on the face of the vast globe; yet medical science has not been able to master the diseases that beset mankind everywhere. Its body of knowledge is large and universal, yet man is not rid of his diseases[186]. The situation is that man still has his incurable diseases, and medicine stands helplessly looking on. Without the use of medicine the Art of Reishi is applied, and before this power all irregularity of physical or mental functioning must disappear. Not even the touch of a finger is required to cure disease: only the transmission of the Internal Action of Reishi. Life is the most precious of all things to man. What will a man take in exchange for his life? Is not the perpetual struggle of man against disease an answer to this question? The last enemy that shall be destroyed is death! The application of the Internal Action of Reishi is the only answer to this question of health; and it is a satisfactory answer.

---

[185] Similar to Usui's words in the Hikkei: 'Our therapy is a spiritualistic method of therapy that has transcended modern science.'

[186] Similarly, Dr Sen Nagai in Usui's Hikkai sats, 'Although I understand the nature of the illness, I do not know how to cure it.'

Once both the External and the Internal Action of Reishi have been mastered there is no further difficulty in being to others the blessing that they require. The practitioner is master over his own illness as well as over those of others. The next chapter will show just how the Internal Action of Reishi may be applied to various diseases in order to render an effective cure, whereby the practitioner may heal his own as well as the disease of others.

WE believe that the will and
function of a community are
fulfilled in accordance with a
spiritual law of rhythm.

Cure of Bad Habits by the Reishi Method

1. Introductory

There are various kinds of evil habits for which there has been found no cure by moralists and physicians of the mind and character. These habits are verily diseases beyond the healing of medical science. Such habits are not only painful and often fatal to those afflicted with them, but exert a baneful influence on society in general. To have found a way of curing such habits is to have found a way of contributing greatly to the reformation and general improvement of human society. This is just what TAIREIDO does. By the application of the Art of Reishi all forms of evil habit can be removed and the moral and physical condition resd to normality.

It is much more difficult to cure a bad habit than to remedy a disease, though in the application of Reishi the methods of treatment are not very different. In the removal of bad habits the period of recovery can be reckoned much in the same way as in removal of disease, though the possibility of certainty as to time is more difficult than in judging of disease. One of the difficulties in eradicating bad habits is that the victims are not conscious of them to the same degree as are people afflicted with bodily ailments. People are far more discriminating in regard to their diseases than in regard to their moral failings. But no matter how reticent or how diffident the victim of bad habits is, the application of the Art of Reishi will res normal conditions or create new and proper conditions if proper treatment be adopted.

The cause of bad habits is usually due to the perversion or abuse of some mental or physical function, either intentionally or through unnatural development. The resulting discordant condition leads to improper habits of mind and body or both. The application of the Action of Reishi to such disordered conditions of mind and body ress the derangement to a natural order and leaves no further cause for the propensity to evil. With the restoration of natural and regular development the bad habits are completely cured.

2. Process of Cure

In the eradication of bad habits, whether physical or mental, the adoption of the Reiyu method is of great value, together with the proper use of the pressure method of finger or palm, as well as the stressed finger and massage methods. It is very important that the agent should exercise the Reiyu method with special reference to the case under treatment, keeping in mind the idea of eliminating the bad habit, though such use of the mind is unnecessary in treating ordinary disease. In case of stammering, for instance, the agent should keep before him the aim of the treatment, namely, to remove the stammering of the patient; and in the case of a victim of alcohol to remove the unnatural desire for intoxicants. If the agent does not maintain a clear conception of the cure that has to be affected, his power in applying the Reishi treatment will be diminished. He must apply the treatment boldly and simply and without confusion of mind[187].

Stammering

To cure stammering in others, which is one of the most obstinate of bad habits, one should bear in mind that there are two forms of this trouble, both of which are equally hard to deal with. One kind of stammering is congenital, and the other due to causes after birth. The latter arises chiefly from imitation. Both of these habits are amenable to Reishi treatment and a cure may assuredly be affected.

First the person that stammers must be made to bring the diaphragm to full tension, standing properly erect, with the eyes and mouth closed. Then with the stressed finger the Internal Action of Reishi should be applied to the

---

[187] Dr Usui's Hikkei suggests similar to the previous three sentences: 'Simply, if the patient suffers pain in the chest, the practitioner of this therapy considers the patient's chest, if the stomach gives pain, then the stomach, and if there is something wrong with the eyes, then the practitioner must be concerned with the patient's eyes themselves'

mouth of the patient, the massage method to the larynx, the stomach and the bowels; after which both pressure and massage should be applied to the head, as in the case of treatment for brain trouble. The agent should finally exercise the Reiyu method with a strong mental effort to remove the trouble. The habit may be cured by one treatment, but sometimes it will require several.

In applying the Reishi treatment the patient should not be made to think too much about it, especially about the method of application, as he is likely to do if he finds the case does not respond quickly to treatment. He must be assured that all cases do not respond with equal freedom and promptness. Without any undue concern as to the outcome the patient should be asked to submit to the treatment regularly until cured. The patient should be taught to practice regularly the deep breathing process, as directed by the Reishi system, so as to strengthen the diaphragm muscles and gain freedom from the Action of Reishi. Whether the patient is gaining such strength from deep breathing may be tested by looking him in the face. If the eyes cannot bravely and fearlessly meet yours the abdomen is weak.

Finger Cramp

This may be a disease sometimes, rather than a habit, but it may here be treated under the caption of habits. It may arise from too much labor at copying or writing; an often musicians, tailors and cigarette maker are victims of it, the trouble usually being in the thumb, forefinger and middle finger. When the trouble is acute the fingers are quite useless.

To cure the affliction by the Reishi system the head of the patient should first be subjected to the same treatment as for brain trouble; and then massage method be applied to the hand and finally the Reiyu method should be adopted. Testing the degree of recovery requires the use of a pen. Then try writing with a brush.

Smoking and Drinking Cramps

The first need of the habitual smoker and drinker is to gain self-control. The tobacco and liquor should be given up at once; for it is very difficult to bring the Action of Reishi to bear on any patient under the influence of tobacco or alcohol, or indeed any kind of drug or poison. This is especially the case if drinking or smoking be to excess. Sometimes these habits are cured simply by application of the Reiyu method, while the victims of the habit are unconscious of the treatment. This is not the ordinary way of curing such habits by the Reishi method, however.

In order to curb the habit of smoking or drinking by the Reishi method the patient must be made to stand in a proper posture and close the eyes and mouth. Then the stressed finger method should be applied to the mouth, the pressure or massage method to the larynx and the stomach and bowels, and the same methods to the head; after which the agent applies the Reiyu method, exercising a strong intention towards cure.

Erotic mania

One of the most terrible habits of men is excessive sexual passion, which sometimes drives the victims to folly if not complete madness. The more excessive is the passion the more difficult it is to cure; but ordinary sexual passion may be easily restrained by application of the Art of Reishi. The ordinary case is due to insufficiency of sexual intercourse; and extreme cases are satisfied with nothing less than a different victim every time.

In treating cases of this kind the pressure method should be applied to the head and to parts of the stomach and bowels; and then the Reiyu method should be applied to the whole body of the patient. It must be remembered that victims of this habit do not usually apply for treatment, except under another name for their trouble. But the agent will usually understand when treating certain diseases that the evil habit is present and must be included in the treatment, either in the presence of the patient or at a distance.

It is well when treating victims of passion to make them practice deep breathing regularly and gain full self-control. Also they should be required to read the biography of noble men and of saintly characters. The patient should be required to abstain from alcohol, tobacco and fatty foods.

Shyness

The habit of experiencing excessive bashfulness or timidity[188] in the presence of superiors or before the public in any capacity is one that should be overcome. Such persons blush too easily; and the head becomes overheated, with consequent trembling and fear; so that both vision and speech are interrupted. In extreme cases there is fainting. The victim usually recovers rapidly from embarrassment on being removed from the occasion of it. It is not unlike nervous debility, though the patient does not usually suffer from that malady.

To cure excessive shyness the patient should be made to take proper posture and bring the diaphragm to full tension. Then apply to the head, breasts and

---

[188] Timidity is given as a condition Reiki may help in Usui's Hikkei

parts of the stomach and bowels and also to the heart the pressure and massage methods; after which exercise the Reiyu method.

The patient should be taught deep breathing in accordance with the Reishi method; and should be advised to read books about heroes and great men, and take plenty of exercise and maintain a cheerful state of mind.

Thievery and Gambling

This from a depravity often displays itself in early life, during boyhood and girlhood, and the danger from it was never more obvious than today. Most of the arrests on this charge are of young persons, some of whom have already acquired the evil practice, the casuals being usually few. The evil is not always due to a naturally avaricious mind but to simple habit.

Few victims of such bad habits apply for treatment; but they may be effectively treated at a distance by the Reishi method, on the request of those interested in their welfare, or they may sometimes be treated while undergoing treatment for some other trouble. In any case the most effective form of Reishi treatment is the Reiyu method.

Women and others, however, who have such habits as shoplifting, should in addition be treated for nervous debility and hysteria or mania.

Patients undergoing treatment for the above habits should be induced to refrain from reading fiction and literature tending to excite the mind or lead one astray.

Gluttony and Ostentation

These bad habits are usually found more commonly among members of the upper classes, though even the more humble members of society may be so afflicted. Gluttony is mostly a habit of man, and ostentation usually a weakness of women. But Epicureanism and vanity alike lead to ruin.

In treating such weakness the Reiyu method is best, as the victims are not gluttons by physical necessity but simply by habit. The habit of ostentation, likewise, is done more to habit than to physical desire for vain display. In some cases application of the Reiyu method at once diminishes the habit and soon removes it completely. In treating such weaknesses care must be taken not to let the patient fall into another bad habit while curing him from the one with which he was first afflicted.

Victims of the above affliction should be advised to abstain from reading exciting or vain books, indeed any kind of literature that appeals to the appetite and to the love of display. The patient should have the mind turned to the common things of life, exercising full control over mind and eye.

Over-cleanliness

To be too scrupulous about cleanliness of person and environment is, and evil peculiar to the Japanese, where bathing is a daily practice and cleanliness a religion. Such habits are taken as a sign of high class associations. But even a good custom can be corrupted. With many people in Japan the time devoted to bathing and toilet is due to a bad habit, which is only a good habit driven to excess.

To cure this habit the Reiyu method should be applied strongly yet without coming in contact with the patient. If, however the patient should be under treatment for some other trouble at the same time, the pressure or the massage method must be applied in addition. Otherwise nothing more is necessary besides the Reiyu method.

To Cure Bad Habits[189] at a Distance[190]

Bad habits of any kind can be cured at a distance just the same as diseases or ailments of the body or mind, the methods being exactly the same in either case. To affect a cure in the absence[191] of the patient the practitioner simply places the photograph[192] or the handwriting of the person to be treated before him and keeps in mind the essential details of the written application. Then he applies the Reiyu method for about five minutes at each treatment. There should be no disappointment, however, if bad habits do not respond to treatment as readily as diseases. It is especially necessary that those undergoing treatment at a distance should not give way to suspicion or doubt if the process prove more slow than they expected. When the patient is at a distance there is not the same opportunity for consultation and advice, which often retards the effectiveness of the process. Personal treatment is preferable where possible. But distance should not lead a patient to suppose that he cannot be successfully treated by the Reishi method; for though it is often more difficult to effect a cure under such circumstances, the cure can be affected nevertheless, if the treatment is properly applied and properly received. There must be freedom to respond and freedom to receive as well as a readiness to persevere on both sides.

---

[189] Dr Usui's Hikkei also mentions the ability of Reiki to help bad habits

[190] Nowadays called 'distant healing'

[191] Nowadays called 'absent healing'

[192] Photographs are often used by modern practitioners of Reiki

Both the agent and the patient should have a clear understanding as to what has to be done.

THE END

TAIREIDO

I

A SYSTEM OF NEW THOUGHT

1. A New Idea

The System of Thought and Life known as TAIREIDO is the most original and effective ever revealed to the mind of man. It has come into the life and thought of Japan like a new revelation and now has far-reaching influence throughout the Empire. It is a Power giving rise to a movement for the complete, reconstruction of civilization: to regenerate nations, society, politics, finance, industry, religion, art, morals, the thought and tendency of the age, and all that pertains to social phenomena. The Power and Direction of the thought and movement is REI, or Spirit, obedience to which brings about a new world.

The fundamental basis of this new system of thought is TAIREIDO, or the Way of the Great Spirit, a new and original evolution of thought, quite independent of any other thought system known to man, and developed from the mind of Mr. Morihei Tanaka, of Tokyo[193], Japan. Though no more than three years[194] have elapsed since this new revelation came to Mr. Tanaka the new doctrine has been quickly taken up by people everywhere and the disciples of TAIREIDO now number thousands[195]. For so brief a time the spread of the new system has been nothing less than marvellous, on

[193] Like Tanaka, Usui was from Tokyo, and may have known each other. As they were both well known, and doing similar work, it is very likely they met. For example, when Sweeney was busiest, he met most leading masters of his day.

[194] Which puts this article date to around 1908.

[195] It is highly likely Usui at least knew of Tanaka's system, because many of Tanaka's 1000s of students practiced in Tokyo in the years before Usui-sensei first used Reiki.

account of the fervent devotion of its followers and ardent zeal of their propaganda.

2. Wonderful Art of Reishi

REISHI is the power of the Great Spirit, TAIREI, in action. TAIREI is not taught simply as a system of thought: it is the spirit or life at the centre of all thought and life. The method of applying this force to life is called Reishi-jutsu, or the Art of the Practice of Reishi. This spirit-action is the source of all life and power in the universe: the essence of existence. To appreciate it and to be able to apply it one must be familiar with the science of Reiri-gaku, the method by which the action of the Spirit manifests itself in matter, to understand which is to apprehend how every phenomenon originates in and proceeds from REISHI, or the Spirit in Action. This new science reveals many truths so wonderful as to seem quite miraculous to those who study the Art of Reishi, explaining even what science has failed to elucidate. The Art of the Practice of Reishi reveals the secrets of all wonders recorded in the past, the mystical phenomena mentioned in the writings of the ancient philosophers and sages, such as the healing of disease by communion with the Divine and the laying on of hands[196], how mind can work upon matter and so on. What the wise men of the past saw but faintly after long years of study, research and experience can now be clearly revealed by no more than ten days training and initiation[197] in the principles and rules pertaining to the Art of Reishi as taught by Mr. Morihei Tanaka. This ten days instruction can be received without any inconvenience to the pupil; there are no ascetic practices required, no painful endeavors necessary: it is open to all who desire it on the same terms, even without prayer or any system of mental concentration. One may be made familiar with the marvellous functions of the Great Spirit, or TAIREI, simply by coming under the instruction offered by Mr. Tanaka, the founder of TAIREIDO. For those who by reason of distance or otherwise are prevented from being present at the lectures given by Mr. Tanaka, there is the volume known as TAIREIDO[198], being a transcript of the lectures of the founder on the subject of practicing the Art of Reishi, which gives a simple and lucid account of the science and its mysteries. Being a divine art, indeed for the good of all mankind, REISHI offers no difficulty of apprehension when once the system is fully

---

[196] Usui's Hikkei mentions the laying on of hands

[197] This suggests training was the equivalent of 5 weekends, and that an initiation (attunement??) took place.

[198] This volume is included within this book

explained: it comes to every mind as a manifestation clear as the sunlight. No human being on realizing the workings of the Art of Reishi can fail to perceive something really miraculous or supernatural, and yet nothing that is not truly natural to Reishi.

3. How the Art of Reishi was Revealed

One of the most interesting and important aspects of the new system of thought and life is the way in which Mr. Tanaka first became conscious of the science of the Art of Reishi, as a bodily experience which he was able to reveal to others and teach them also to experience. This power to let others into the apparent secret of the Art of Reishi, and how he came to feel it incumbent on him to transmit the wonderful power he had become aware of, the reader may discover by pursuing the following pages.

The founder of TAIREIDO had always been a man deeply moved by patriotic enthusiasm. When the Liaotung peninsula was ceded to Japan at the close of the war with China the whole nation rejoiced with patriotic ardor; but when Japan was forced to relinquish the fruit of her victory through the intervention of three Powers the retrocession brought tears to every Japanese eye. After this humiliation it soon became clear that Russia was pursuing a policy of aggression in East Asia, for she took advantage of the Boxer Rebellion to send large numbers of Troops into China controlling the railways and erecting barracks which betrayed intentions of permanent occupation of the territory. China later obtained from Russia consent to a treaty of evacuation, and the principle of the 'open door', but Russia failed to live up to the terms of the Agreement, and in 1903 Russia did not hesitate to announce her intentions to remain in Manchuria for good. Accordingly she established a Far Eastern regime under a Governor-General, Alexief being the first to hold office, an incarnation of Russian jingoism. To Alexief the Tsar granted supreme power in the Far East, and he took command of Russian diplomacy and military matters. Thus the promise to evacuate Manchuria and to observe the principle of the 'open door' was absolutely ignored by Russia, and the other Powers were practically given to understand that Russia intended permanently to occupy the territory. Japan objected to this aggression on China, but Russia only assured a provocative attitude toward Japan, and the situation soon assumed a threatening aspect in East Asia. At first the attitude of the Japanese authorities toward Russia was rather one of irresolution and indecision, against which inactivity there was loud complaints in Japan where the people insisted that war, was inevitable.

At this very juncture in Japan's foreign relations Mr. Morihei Tanaka was only twenty years of age, and an official in the Government bureau of statistics, attending betimes the School of Foreign Languages. He had been carefully studying the situation in Manchuria and the problem arising out of it, and came to the popular conclusion that there was no way to ensure peace in the Far East save by prompt action on the part of the Government in dealing with Russia. To neglect the matter was to sow seeds of calamity for the future of the Empire. But what could a youth of twenty do under the circumstances? For a time he could do no more than watch with anxiety the increasing war-cloud gathering over the Empire. Unable to restrain his patriotic feelings longer, Mr. Tanaka resolved to act; and to do this in the most emphatic way, he planned the gravest and most imposing of all the methods, a direct appeal to His Majesty the Emperor. Accordingly, when His Majesty was returning to the Imperial Palace after attending the military maneuvers, young Tanaka boldly took his life in his hands and interrupted the Imperial procession to present his appeal to the Emperor.

This ever-memorable day was the 19th of November, 1903. The sky was clear and the autumnal breezes were blowing gently, as His Majesty emerged in the usual imposing procession from Sakurada Gate, when suddenly a youth was seen to rush toward the Imperial carriage, and shouting that he desired to present a petition to the Emperor, he reached the Imperial carriage before any of the guards could stop him, and handed the document to His Majesty. Just as the Emperor glanced at the lad, an official seized him and bore him away under arrest. He had succeeded in presenting his petition, however: and the following is a translation of the now famous document:

"A common citizen of the Empire, Morihei Tanaka by name, most humbly and reverently begs to report to the Imperial Throne, as follows: YOUR MAJESTY, THE EMPEROR, whose civil and military virtues are everywhere renowned, has achieved the Imperial Restoration and brought prosperity to the Empire, for which all subjects are moved to tears of gratitude, and for this gracious Imperial benevolence we desire to make adequate return to Your Majesty. I am persuaded that to establish the Empire on a firm foundation is not more important than to preserve the nation's dignity and right of the nation that enemy should be opposed with all our might. The Manchurian situation now facing us threatens to dishonor the nation and to trespass on the rights of the Empire. Nothing can be more dangerous to Japan than to leave this problem unsolved. Half a year has elapsed since this menace arose, and our Ministers of State ought to have reached a decision long ago; and yet hesitation and indecision mark their course and threaten our future. This is not a time for compromise; peaceful and timid negotiations can never ensure peace to the Far East. Russia has ignored the treaty concluded with China, and any treaty she concludes with Japan will prove a blank page in our history. Yet, we are told, the responsible Ministers are determined to solve the problem peaceably. If this be true, nothing can be more regrettable, for nothing can prevent our national ruin.

What the present situation needs is a decisive attitude; we must be prepared to assert our dominant influence and be ready for the last resort. Unless this be done disorder and not peace will be the lot of East Asia, and the future of our Empire will be very unhappy. All this must be fully known to the subjects of Your Majesty, and even to foreign countries. Failing at this critical moment, the forty millions of Japan and the hundreds of millions in Asia will be threatened. The time-serving peace now suggested by the officials of the Government will bring perpetual unrest to the Far East. The only way to peace is through present war! This is not the only time that our Empire has been dishonored by Russia. Through her we lost Saghalien, and through her we lost the Liaotung peninsula after the war with China; and now Russia is again threatening us with further disgrace and intruding upon our rights. Shall Japan endure this insult or not? If we submit to this nothing can save us in future!

Japan has sufficient defenses if she has but the courage to use them. All we have to do is to act promptly and success is ours. If we fail properly to chastise the enemy now the Empire will lose its dominant influence and fall prey to the Russian eagle. This is the most crucial moment ever reached by the Empire. I humbly beseech and pray that Your Gracious Majesty will issue an edict that we may act upon and save the nation from eternal regret. I, a youth of but twenty years, am compelled by burning patriotism and loyalty in connection with the present unfortunate situation, so that I can neither sleep nor eat, to make this request, I therefore have dared to interrupt the Imperial procession and intrude upon Your August Majesty, thinking of the fate of our Empire and the eight hundred millions of the Orient. May Your Majesty ever continue to grant us enlightenment; and may it please Your Majesty to hear and heed this humble petition from a common citizen, Morihei Tanaka, conveying his sincere solitude for the Empire."

The Imperial History Association, in its history of the Russo-Japanese war, referring to the incident of Morihei Tanaka presenting a petition to the Emperor, says: "The petition this presented to the Throne was quite pertinent to the situation, and was no exaggeration of the national voice. Even youth could not refrain from taking so irregular a step, moved by indignation over the situation. His move was, therefore, approved by the public."

The various references to the incident in the daily press were favorable to the motive of young Tanaka and spoke highly of his zeal and patriotism under the circumstances. He, therefore, received no further punishment than to be sent to his native province for the time being. Thus confined to his native place young Tanaka gave himself up to contemplation, preparing the way for the marvellous revelation of new thought that came to him later.

4. Influence of the Mountains[199]

After young Tanaka was returned to his native place for daring to make a direct report to the Imperial Throne, he was kept under constant surveillance by officers of the law, and his life was practically deprived of freedom. He established himself in a small cottage in the mountain village of Takenami, which he called Somoan. There he put in a time of contrition and patience, giving greater attention to the international problem that had been troubling him and had got him into difficulty. The year 1904 passed without any incident of importance, but relations with Russia were on the verge of rapture. Mr. Tanaka was still greatly disturbed that the authorities still took no decisive step in regard to Russia. But he could do nothing on account of being constantly watched by the police. Before the year was over, however, the outcome was that Mr. Tanaka desired, and the war with Russia began, the first stroke of the fight being the attack on the Russian warships at Chemulpo and Port Arthur. The Imperial declaration of war was at last issued and the whole nation was united as one man to die for the glory of the Empire. In this patriotic enthusiasm Mr. Tanaka duly joined, but as he was under military age he was not allowed to proceed to the front; and in any case being under police surveillance would have prevented it. He could only hope, and pray for victory. At this time we find the following reference to Mr. Tanaka in the *Achi*, a daily newspaper:

Beginning with the heading: Information about the youth who attempted to appeal to the Throne, the article proceeds: "Mr. Tanaka, after being sent to his native place, has been spending his time in penitence and meditation for having offended against the rules pertaining to Imperial processions, and has built himself a small cottage in a mountain village where he does a great deal of reading. On the outbreak of the war he was so delighted that at once he sent off a congratulatory letter to all his friends and acquaintances. In this

[199] Tanaka's story is very similar to the story of Usui's studies and spiritual discipline on Kurama-yama in the mountains of Gifu.

letter were the following words: "In defiance of the Government regulations I dared to appeal directly to the Imperial Throne, blinded by zeal for the good of my country. My delight on hearing that the Imperial Declaration of war had been issued was simply indescribable: I was almost mad with emotion. Now the Imperial army and navy have advanced upon the enemy and victory is reported even from the beginning. A series of victories on the part of the army and the ultimate submission of the enemy may duly be expected. I therefore sincerely offer my congratulations on the proclamation of war by the Empire." Mr. Tanaka is really a man of admirable spirit, most gentle and upright in all his ways, and his assiduous habits of study are the admiration of the officers watching him."

The founder of TAIREIDO thus lived quietly in this mountain retreat for several months, meditating on his condition and on life in general. He came finally to this conclusion: There is no doubt that victory to Japan is certain; but victory over Russia will not be enough; it is after the war that the main difficulty will arise. He foresaw that the ability of Korea and China to maintain independence would be very difficult. To a great extent this would depend on the future of the Japanese Empire. The situation evidently implied that there would be annexations by Japan. Under the influence of such thoughts Mr. Tanaka wrote a long essay on the subject entitled: The Annexation of East Asia, which was published in the *Nihonjin*, the essay incurring the displeasure of the Government, which led to its author being placed under still stricter official surveillance.

In the course of time the character and real motives of Mr. Tanaka became understood by the officials of the Government and he came in for more generous treatment. After gaining further liberty he ascended the sacred mountain of Ena[200], where the Sun Goddess is reputed to have been born, and there for a time he practiced strict religious austerities[201]. This was the turning point in his career. It was then that he first began to realize the meaning of TAIREIDO and to experience the practice of the Art of Reishi. The fundamental Spirit within him then first began to manifest its functions. There in the silent recesses of the great mountains he remained secluded until TAIREIDO became fully revealed to him[202], and he saw that he could solve all the problems of life by virtue of the revelation, even the problems that no metaphysical study could approach.

---

200 Usui-sensei is also said to have ascended a sacred mountain – Kurama.

201 As did Usui-sensei

202 Remarkably similar to how it is thought Reiki was revealed to Usui.

5. Effect of Asceticism

The year 1904 was marked by Japan's victories over Russia, and especially the fall of Port Arthur. When news of this famous victory came it found Mr. Tanaka in the fastness of the mountain, and inspired him with still grander thoughts, to which his sublime surroundings added not a little. He felt a divine enlightenment descend upon him in the sacred mountain where the Sun Goddess shed her divine rays. The great peaks around him soared into the heavens, clothed in mysterious mist; the deep verdure of the lower Altitudes environed him and seemed to shut in secrets never revealed to man. Out of the vast abyss ripping the mountains the key to knowledge was handed to him; as he solemnly took it he could hear only music of the streams in the depths below. The rising sun unclothed the mountain and revealed its true beauty and power. The garments of mist again lifted, the silver light penetrating every crevice and ravine. The birds and insects slept and peace reigned: peace, and power, and beauty! The night dissolved away! All this was in man too: this peace, and power and beauty. Thus Mr. Tanaka meditated in the recesses of the giant hills and communed with the Spirit that produced them, experiencing thoughts and emotions transcending the universe. Thus the Great Spirit, the Spirit of God Almighty expressed itself.

Among the more compelling thoughts of these sublime moments were these: Man is a self-conscious being; he is aware of his own existence. What then is the basis of his life: its real essence? Life is a combination of matter and spirit, of body and mind. Nothing spiritual can exist without its material counterpart, and *vice versa.* Idealism is one side of the shield, and materialism is the reverse side. These are not contrary, the one to the other. The mind and the body mutually exist in each other; and there must be something that is the origin of these. What is that something? What is its fundamental nature and essence? Can man utilize it?

Human life as we know it is maintained by taking food and breathing air; and therefore these two things must contain the essence of man's existence, since on them it mainly depends. Of the two, the air is the more important, for though one can live several days without food, one cannot live even several minutes without air. Air is, therefore, the first element in the maintenance of life; and food comes second. This gave rise to the question of what would be the effect on human life if only air were supplied and food withheld. Would any change be experienced in the mind and in the body? How long can a human being live on the first element essential to his existence, air? To this experiment Mr. Tanaka devoted himself in order to obtain one of the fundamental answers to the problems of life.

He accordingly gave himself up to a period of fasting. The period commenced on the first of February, 1905 and ended at the beginning of June, a space of ninety days, which may be regarded as a record duration in abstention from food. The fasting, however, was the least important part of this experiment; for he experienced spiritual realities beyond all words to describe[203]. The most important of the revelations that then came to him was that concerning the Art of Reishi, the working of the Spirit. He had other mysterious experiences, such as power to see things in the dark, and the ability to run as swiftly as one flying, to see great and unusual distances, and to hear sound far beyond the normal distance.

6. Welcome Home

After a period of some six months solitude in the sacred mountain Mr. Tanaka returned to his native village, the time being about the beginning of July. It was apparent to all his old friends and acquaintances that he was a changed man. His long contemplation in communion with the forces of nature and the wonderful spiritual experiences that came to him during his period of fasting had worked a miraculous effect on him, which all could see. The revelation of TAIREI, its full meaning and significance, had come to him. Not only so, but he had the power to put into practice the truth that was his[204], to the wonder and admiration of all who came in contact with him. His action in irregularly presenting a petition to the Throne had already made him a marked man; but the powers he now revealed in a spiritual way made him far more distinguished among those who knew him. Many gathered around him to hear his experiences and to learn his art. The supreme moment of his realizing the good effect his new knowledge was to have on his fellow men, came just when he heard of the great victory of the Japanese navy over Russia in the battle of the Japan Sea. He said nothing of it until the people began to tell him the news; which was no news to him, as he had realized the truth of it all before. When it became known that he knew of the victory of the battle of the Japan Sea before it was reported in his native village, the thing seemed nothing less than a miracle.

---

[203] All Tanaka's story is remarkably similar to stories of Usui's mountain experience. Usui's Hikkei: 'During my period of fasting, I exposed myself to the atmosphere. In so doing, I was wondrously inspired, and realized purely by chance that I had discovered the spiritual capabilities of therapy.'

[204] Similarly, one story about Usui is that he descended from the sacred mountain and his spiritual experiences, and had the ability to immediately help and heal others with Reiki.

After this he began to feel the Spirit of prophecy; and he began to predict peace with Russia would be resd through the intervention of the President of the United States, with a result disadvantageous to Japan; and the prediction came true. The peace negotiated at Portsmouth resulted just as Mr. Tanaka had foretold. People might think that such predictions were no more than shrewd guesses; but there are facts in relation to Mr. Tanaka that cannot be so regarded. A woman who had suffered from years from rheumatism, on hearing of the powers of Mr. Tanaka, came to him for relief and he completely cured her. Again a girl who suffered from chronic toothache was fully cured by him simply by touching the affected part[205]. These facts the people were obliged to believe because they could not be contradicted. Such miraculous deeds evoked the wonder of the community, and excited the utmost curiosity among the people, until the agent of them began to be visited by people from far and near, all of whom deeply admired his wonderful art.

7. Miraculous Experience while in the Spirit

As already indicated, after his experiences in the mountain, Mr. Tanaka became aware of his possession of more than ordinary powers over nature, enabling him to apprehend the truth of TAIREI and to apply it by means of Reishi to his fellow men. These supernatural functions inherent in the human body first revealed their existence to Mr. Tanaka during the fasting period of his meditation in the mountain; and he was convinced of the power and use of functions which he believed had never before been revealed to man

This power over nature he saw to lie in the command of Rei, or Spirit, the essence on which all life depends. This power it is that causes the ability to think, to will, to decide, to feel, to know, to exercise muscular action and command the action of the body. It is, moreover, the entity on which Creation depends, from which all matter organic and inorganic comes, and the author and giver of life. TAIREIDO is the method by which this essence functions. Even from remote ages it has been admitted that man can somehow come in contact with the essence of things, and touch the mysteries of the universe, and fasting has long been regarded as the gateway to this experience.

---

[205] Usui-sensei was also thought to have come down from the mountain and healed a girl's toothache, and achieved other miraculous healings. There seem to be many 'co-incidences'?

In the Buddhist sutras we read that Amida ate but one grain of hemp seed every day for six years. While the statement is no doubt and exaggeration it is obviously intended to denote the extreme asceticism of the founder of Buddhism before he could achieve his great life purpose and come to his spiritual awakening at the foot of the bo-tree. Jesus Christ was led up of the Spirit to be tempted in the wilderness by the Devil, and there he fasted forty days and forty nights after which he suffered from hunger. He was able to reject the temptations of the evil spirit and to prove himself the Son of God, and the angles ministered to him. After this he did many wonderful things for men. Buddha practiced an ascetic life for six years before he reached the period of his awakening, though he partook of some food; and Jesus attained his awakening after forty days and nights of fasting, but Mr. Tanaka fasted ninety days, which is unprecedented; yet all agree in the conviction that by fasting and meditation the highest enlightenment can be attained. The teachings of such sages as Buddha and Christ have prevailed widely since their death; but they left the world without showing the secret of their achievements. Man has not learned the way to command over the powers of nature. He has seen wonderful deeds but has not acquired the art of doing them. The sages have shown the way of prayer and taught the benefit of self-denial in order to reach spiritual enlightenment and awakening; but the founder of TAIREIDO has achieved quite a different triumph. He has acquired not only the secret of command over nature and man but also the ability to impart this gift to man, even through his ten days′ instruction in the elements of TAIREIDO, to all who desire to receive such knowledge.

The best way for beginners, instead of taking up at first a technical study of TAIREIDO, is to attend the lectures of Mr. Tanaka[206] and see this wonderful power practiced before their eyes, so as to be convinced of its truth and reality. This can be done any time at the headquarters of the office of TAIREIDO, where the Art of Reishi is constantly seen in practice.

At these lectures Mr. Tanaka usually begins by giving a careful explanation of the way of meditation to all present. Only fifty persons are permitted to attend each lecture, as they must always sit in the rows. It will be interesting if we describe the scene at one of these lectures. When the instruction begins there is a stillness that is breathless. One can almost hear the throbbing of his neighbor's heart. Mr. Tanaka appears and stands in the midst of the hall, and at once begins to transmit to those present the force of

---

[206] It is suggested by some that soon after his mountain enlightenment, Usui also gave many lectures.

Rei.[207] There is at once a stillness and solemnity like unto the depths of a great forest. This quietness is the centre of a spiritual typhoon which is nevertheless airless. But the stillness is but the foretaste of something better still, something very unusual that strangely looms upon the vision of all present.

The hand of the clock covers one minute, two minutes, three minutes, when a gentle tremor is experienced by the audience. After a brief space one of the members of the class in front begins to show violent physical perturbation in the way of a tremor, which seems to affect his neighbors, and soon all those present feel similar pulsations, until a commotion of some violence takes place. The body moves up and down, then to right and left, now forward and backward; and everyone feels that something very marvellous has been experienced. What is the secret of this violent surging and moving within the body of each one present? After a period the audience recovers its former quiet and stillness. Then the tremor is repeated and the same commotion takes place again. The tremor imparted to the whole class is thus repeated five times or so, taking some twenty minutes; and then the instructor announces the end of his first lecture and practice of the Art of Reishi.

8. First Step in Acquiring the Art of Reishi

The first step in acquiring the art of Reishi is experiencing the tremor of the Spirit described in the preceding paragraph. Within the body and spirit of man there is the Action of the Spirit, or Reishi, the origin and essence of life and being. The form by which it manifests its presence is known as the revelation of Reishi in action. To bring this about this manifestation all the members of the class in the room are made to stand and take hands; whereupon Mr. Tanaka, taking his place in the circle, and holding hands of those on either side of him, at once transmits the Action of Reishi to the whole circle[208]. The hands which he touches begin to reveal the tremor of the Action and move to and for, until the motion circulates through the class. Sometimes this motion grows so intense that the individuals of the circle jump as high as eight inches from the floor and some even as high as from one to two feet. When all are thus affected they are required to release hands and drop them by the sides and the motion ceases. As the jumping is straight up without bending the knees or legs it is clearly not intentional but the result of the Action of Reishi alone. All are not affected just the same, and

---

[207] This is how modern Reiki seminars may work.

[208] A version of Mawashi, as taught by Hiroshi Doi in Japan and Sweeney

when any individual shows a tendency to be too slow he is assisted by just a touch from the hand of Mr. Tanaka, when he will at once respond to the Action of Reishi, by violently jumping.

9. Transmitting Reishi Action to groups or Numbers

In commencing instruction Mr. Tanaka usually first transmits the Action of Reishi to individuals, and after they have acquired the art of receptivity he transmits the Action to groups thus first instructed individually. By having been taught in this preliminary manner how to receive the Action of Reishi they naturally respond readily in group action. When groups are fully under the influence of the Reishi Action the jumping is so violent that the room resounds with their commotion. An interesting feature of these lessons in the transmission of the Action of Reishi is the fact that so long as Mr. Tanaka remains in contact with the group circle the Action of Reishi in them is strong even to violence, but as soon as he releases contact with the circle the Action of Reishi perceptibly weakens[209].

This movement of the body resulting from the transmission of the Action of Reishi is fundamental to the method by which human life and health are strengthened and improved in the briefest space of time. *A few minutes practice of this Art of Reishi several times a day will soon res one's health, promote physical robustness and develop the natural beauty of the body, eliminating all disease.*

10. How to Apprehend the Meaning of the Action of Reishi

The mental and spiritual process involved in receiving the thought and action of another is something too wide for discussion here, but the popular conception of it is that the thought in A's mind becomes the action in B's mind; or in other words, B acts what A thinks, when their hands are in contact. This method has been at time practiced in western countries too[210].

But the art of apprehending what is in the mind of others is not the highest development of the Action of Reishi; yet it is none the less very interesting and of much benefit to those studying the Art of the Action of Reishi. This art is specially taught by Mr. Tanaka as conductive to a more apt and intelligent apprehension of Reishi in Action. It is an art that can be readily acquired and practiced by anyone who has studied the internal Action of Reishi.

---

209 Perhaps an example of Tanaka's mastery

210 Theosophy teachings also had such conceptions and the theosophist H.S. Olcott visited Japan as early as 1889.

The student begins by practicing the Art through hand contact, and when successful in this way, he is moved on to a higher way. The contact of hands might be supposed to have some hint of the thought passing in the mind of another, and thus suggestion might pass from A to B; and moreover, as any change in the manner, such as grasping the hand lightly or tightly might tend to confusion or distraction in the case of those not fully acquainted with the Art of Reishi Action, a higher form of the experiment has been introduced.

By this method and individual is placed between the agent who thinks and the agent who is to receive and act on the thought, so that the thought has to be transmitted through a second party to the third party, who is to act upon it. After succeeding in transmission of thought by this means a third, fourth and fifth intermediary are introduced between the transmitter and receiver. Mr Tanaka is the only agent that has ever succeeded in this complex method of thought transmission. As the intermediaries between A and B do not know what is in the mind of A, and have no idea of the thought transmitted, they do not cause any confusion in the mind of B, and this B apprehends the thought of A without any hint or suggestion form any source. Four gentlemen notably successful in this action are Mr. Asataro Sakurai, Mr. Mikitaro Iijima, Mr. Sekita Oyama and Mr. Shosuke Ikeda. These have been able to transmit thought by every combination of their number, acting as A and B. Those who have witnessed the phenomenon of mind-reading will have noticed that it is always done in a solemn and grave manner that tends to make one smile. To anyone the scene is something to excite the most profound interest, quite beyond words to describe.

For example, six men are placed in a line, with hands in contact. The man at the left of the row of men becomes the thought-transmitter, A; and A secretly determines who of the number is to become the receiver of his thought and lets the individual know. None of the others are aware of the decision. Then 'A' concentrates his thought on what he wants his agent to do and the agent does what A decides. All having their eyes closed except A. In practicing this experiment the thought of A must be firm and clear; but B, the receiver, need not have any special state of mind or will. The receiver, or mind-reader, stands at the right side, or end of the row, with all the others between him and A, the transmitter. We have seen this experiment successfully practiced with seven men in the row. During the experiment the following results were obtained:

1. B went into another room and brought out a chair; 2. He place the chair before the Altar of Rei, the Great Spirit; 3. He brought a cushion from the corner of the room, dropping it and picking it up on the way; 4. He went to

the office and summoned Mr. Fujimoto who was attending his duty and unaware of the experiment three rooms away; 5. He asked him to sit on the chair; 6. He brought in the tea things from the servant's room; 7. He took up a cup and handed it to Mr. Tanaka; 8. He then poured out a cup of tea in the proper manner and quantity; 9. He replaced the teapot on the tray; 10. He put his hand on that of Mr. Fujimoto and assisted him to raise the teacup to his mouth.

The above actions were done by B in the most offhand manner without mistakes, his eyes closed from beginning to end. The success of such an experiment in such complex action depended on the clearness and strength of A's mind in transmitting his thought to B. In such a case B acts strictly in accord with A's thought. It will be noticed that B dropped the cushion when bringing it into the room; this was due to the determination of the agent that this action should happen by B's losing the Action of Reishi for the moment. At this moment Mr. Tanaka, was standing apart from the line of men. But B promptly picked up the dropped cushion by stopping; which was also part of Mr. Tanaka's predetermined thought. Thus Mr. Tanaka by the Art of Reishi was able to interfere between A and B and cause B to drop the cushion and pick it up again, neither A nor B being privy to his intention. This proves that B was influenced by an agent outside the row through which the Action of Reishi was being transmitted, because the art of Mr. Tanaka was so powerful. Now all this Action of Reishi, which seems so mysterious in this experiment, is nevertheless being unconsciously practiced by everyone in daily life; which fact shows that no particular study is required in order to be able to utilize the art in a special manner for higher purposes.

Take another example. Make seven men stand in a row and cause the Action of Reishi to circulate violently through them, all going round with the action. In this experiment the transmitter was able to cause the receiver of the thought to bring a man into the room and have him stand there; to bring in another man and have him stand beside the first one; in all seven men were brought in; then he caused the seven men to take hands; then he made the first man take the hand of the seventh man to form a circle; and then he caused them all to go around in a ring. While this experiment may seem rather simple, it was not so easy to make the men go around rapidly in a circle, as was done in this case. To be able to receive the thought transmitted in a definite manner and quickly to transmute it into action without mistake is not as easy as it may seem; yet it has been practiced with complete success. Such an experiment is quite an easy one for a master like Mr. Tanaka; but in the case above mentioned it was accomplished for the first time by members of his class in the Art Reishi of Action.

A further example consists in taking a sheet of paper from a certain room and placing it on the table in the practicing room, and then causing the receiver to go again to the first room and bring a brush for writing, dip it in the ink and cause the holder to write a word or ideograph. This experiment was successfully practiced through the medium of six men. In this case B under the influence of A's mind went into another room which was three rooms distant; took a piece of paper on the table there; returned to the practicing room with it; placed it on the table; went back to the room; took a writing brush and dipped it in the ink; brought it to the practicing room; and wrote the ideograph desired.

Though this experiment also looks simple it is nevertheless quite difficult. A Belgian scientist, Dr. Johann, who saw this experiment, thought the most difficult part of it for thought transmission was the writing of the ideograph by the art of Reishi, especially as the eyes of B were quite closed. But B's consciousness has nothing to do with what he does; he is wholly under the influence of A. The relation between A and B is not the relation of mind and body; it is closer than that, a fusion of minds for the moment. But B cannot always act as A wants him to; for the fusion of thought is not so perfect as to be a fusion of mind. When 'A' thinks of a certain ideograph, say the figure one, he determines that B shall write that character. If A wants to have B write a dash or a line it is not so difficult for the action is one merely of space and time; but for a more complicated figure, the mind of A has to concentrate on when the writing brush must be applied and when it must be withheld, through every movement necessary, since the action is not the action of B's mind at all but of A's mind, B having really no mind but A's for the time being. The figure reproduced here is taken directly from the one written by B at the instance of A under the Action of Reishi. In such a proceeding, speaking strictly, B does not know that he is acting at the instance of A, or that he has a brush in his hand at all. The whole process is due to the power of A's mind over B.

The above experiments will show some aspects of the power of Reishi once one has acquired the Art of using it. It is not the art of thought transmission by contact of hands or other physical method of suggestion, as it is done without such means. Neither is it a system of hypnotism; for this requires entire abstraction of mind on the part of B. The Art of Reishi requires connection between the mind of 'A' and the body of B resulting in action on the part of the latter. It differs from hypnotism in that in the Art of Reishi A does not appropriate the consciousness of B. The only explanation is that Rei, the essence of being, causes the action desired. Consequently the power manifested in this action is the same as that manifested in the usual Action of Reishi, as when the agent has the power to cure sickness or disease at a distance from the patient.

> WE believe that *Reishi* manifests itself in a form of action symbolically represented by the sign 卍; and that the alternation of all transient phenomena in the world is the very action of *Reishi* itself.

II

Art of Thought Transmission

Makes Remarkable Progress

1. Result on Social Life

The term, Thought Transmission, does not quite accurately denote what the Art means, but the meaning thereby conveyed is as near as human language can probably approach it[211].

When the boy is under the power of the mind man is said to lead a conscious existence; but when one's body is governed by the will of another and acts accordingly, there is present the Art of Reishi, as seen to some extent in daily life. All the social activities of mankind are but the result of the automatic action of Reishi, which is fully explained in the volume on the doctrines, principles and teaching of TAIREIDO. As human society is the result of the mechanical action of Reishi all of us are more or less unconsciously under the will of others in thought and action. A man's mind and body are even in close relationship; and it is, therefore, but natural that an expert in the Art of Reishi shall be able quickly to receive what is in the mind of another or others and act accordingly. The practice of the Art as

---

[211] Modern organizations employing Reiki therapists, e.g. surgery, hospital or health research project, are not usually enamored to see 'psychic' therapist. Modern Reiki healers do better to separate their healing abilities totally from any potential they have for being psychic – even to have two business cards if necessary, one as a therapist, and one as a psychic?

seen at the initiation meetings of TAIREIDO students is not simply a manifestation of remarkable spiritual phenomena; for the members present physically experience the Action of the will of others on them; and this proves the possibility of using such action for the welfare of society. To accept the outward manifestation of will is merely to lose one's own individuality; but to understand a proper use of this power by the Art of Reishi gives one a spiritual strength and steadiness that are necessary for true life. To be firm and steadfast in life one must know the power of mind over matter, of spirit over body, both in regard to oneself and to others. In this way one knows the truth and can penetrate into the essential nature of human society. This is what TAIREIDO does for man. It gives him the knowledge and the power necessary to enable him to maintain his own individuality and at the same time to adapt himself in the best way to the needs of society. He is susceptible to all influence and has the power to decide what he shall submit to. Such principles of TAIREIDO as that of maintaining inflexibility of spirit and individual self-respect indicate what a man must be susceptible to, and the principles of adaptation to change show how he must meet the negative aspects of life. Thus the thoughts and principles involved in TAIREIDO touch the loftiest altitudes and the profoundest depths of existence, at the same time showing how they may be practically applied to daily life. This is possible through marvels of the Action of Reishi, which enables man to put into practice the principles revealed in the Action of Reishi.

2. Fuller Development of the Art of Reishi

After gaining complete experience in the art of transmitting thought by the action of Reishi the student goes on to a fuller acquirement of the principles of TAIREIDO. The student already understands how thought is transmitted by contact of hands, then by direct action of the mind of A on the body of B without physical contact, with several individuals between, or even with no more than a string between them. Having perceived how the Action of Reishi may be apprehended and appropriated the student should proceed to fuller knowledge and practice of TAIREIDO, in which so many have attained great success.

At the thirtieth lecture of Mr. Tanaka on the Art of Apprehending the Action of Reishi, this spring, proof of remarkable progress in the knowledge of TAIREIDO was given by some practical experiments. At a similar meeting held in February, 1919, the photograph shown here was taken. First the common method of apprehending what is in the mind of another was practiced by joining hands. At the meeting in the spring the experiment was tried of having A and B stand some twenty feet apart with a string between them. This experiment was a complete success. A desired B to bring a chair, to select a certain individual from a group, to fetch him, to make him sit down on the chair; and all the actions were carried out without mistake. In this experiment Mr. Hakurei Kurihara acted as A and Mr. Shinji acted as B, Mr.Kawaimei Kinoshita being the individual selected to sit on the chair.

Another interesting experiment at this meeting was to place six persons between A and B, these knowing nothing of what A intended to transmit to B; and yet B acted wholly in accord with the mind of A without variation. In this experiment B went and brought three cushions, placed them correctly, selected one of the guests present and had him sit on one of the cushions, brought in the tea things from a table in another room, poured out tea in a cup and gave it to the guest on the cushion: all was done exactly as Mr. Tanaka, who acted as A, had determined mentally. In this experiment Mr. Kenzo Sugizaki was the agent acted upon by Mr. Tanaka, while Mr. Matsusaburo hino was the gentleman acting as the guest.

These successes achieved in the art of transmitting and apprehending thought by the Art of Reishi were achieved by the persons named after only ten days instruction in the art from Mr. Tanaka. So astonished were these pupils at what they had received from Mr. Tanaka's teaching that they thought it nothing less than miraculous.

At a special lecture given by Mr. Tanaka in March 1919, some 26 persons submitted to experiment, when A at one end of the row, and B at the other, succeeded in transmission and apprehension of thought without difficulty or mistake.

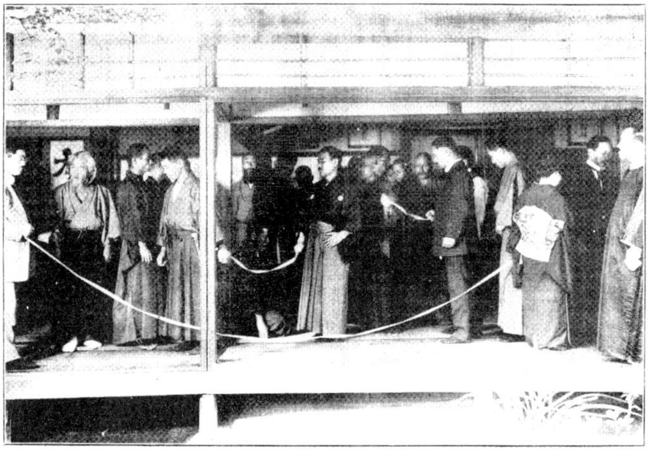

TRANSMITTING REISHI ACTION TO GROUPS

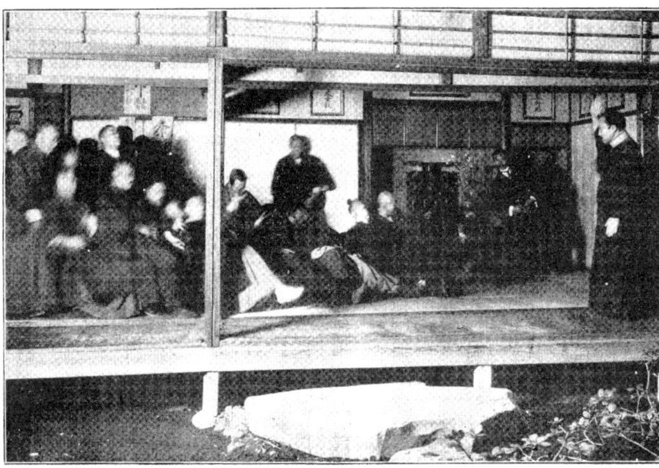

CAUSING A GROUP TO FALL DOWN BY THE POWER OF REISHI

This experiment was different from all preceding ones in that the transmitter wanted to transmit his thought to all of the 25 men. The thought was this. A transmitted to the last man in the row the thought to leave the row and proceed around the class from the inside, and then he transmitted to the next last man the same idea, and so the same idea to all in turn until reaching himself; and thus the whole class of 25 men was set moving in a circle, A concentrating his thought now on the men until finally they were all like a solid ball unable to move, save in violent whirling motion, the man in the centre being so pressed by the others that he went up in the air screaming as if from suffocation.

3. Practicing the Art over a Distance

At the thirty-third meeting for instruction to students of TAIREIDO great interest was taken by the members in some new experiments in transmission of thought at greater distances. No connection at all was permitted between the transmitter and the receiver of thought. The thought in A's mind was that B should put on his hat, take his cane and walk three times around a pine tree near the entrance to the chamber, and stand by the stone step and strike it seven times. B did all this exactly as 'A' wished[212]. The next experiment consisted in A desiring a chair to be brought and placed before the altar of Rei, to have a guest sit on it, to bring in the tea utensils and to offer the guest tea: all of which was accurately done by B as shown in the illustration. In this photograph Mr. Yosaburo Honda is acting as A and Lady Masago Yui as B. Then Mr. Honda decided by thought transmission to have B take a pot of chrysanthemum from an outer chamber, hold it for a time, pass along the path before the chamber, enter the garden facing the lecture room, and stand on the stone step; all of which was being accurately done, when the photograph reproduced was taken. After the picture was taken B came down from the stone step, placed the flower pot on the veranda and did all that A had planned. After this experiment was thus successfully completed Mr. Honda decided to act on Mr. Yui, whom he caused by mental action to proceed slowly along until he passed by the pine tree, reached the gate, stooped down and picked up five pebbles, returned along the same path, came to the entrance and entered, laid the pebbles on the left side of the room, just as Mr. Honda had decided. All this time Mr. Honda was standing at the entrance, the space between them at times being over hundred feet; but distance seemed to have no weakening effect on the power of B to apprehend the thought of A. This was a record-breaking experience in the TAIREIDO class. In all this operation the eyes of B were quite closed, yet in none of the complex actions performed, such as the picking up of pebbles and returning to the house, there was not the slightest mistake made. B did not even stumble as he stepped over stones and went out to the street. It was evident that this action A's eyes must have been used by B.

---

[212] Students who wish to practice this, should only do so with friends who agree to the experiment, otherwise it could be termed an abuse of power.

4. Art of Self Defense by Reishi

The art of overcoming others by Reishi has also been successfully practiced by students of TAIREIDO[213]. Some interesting experiments in this art were successfully carried out at the meeting referred to in the foregoing paragraph. A determined to practice on B; and was so successful that simply by holding out his hand A made B fall to the ground like a stick, or like a tree when felled. At one meeting when sixty members practiced this art the scene was a most lively and interesting one. Members that began to practice as A next time acted as B, and were acted upon with complete success. It took but a short time for all the students to become familiar with the art. After the art of throwing an individual by Reishi is understood the student next tries to hand at throwing groups, when 'A' holds out his hand and exerts the internal action of Reishi and all the members of the group at once fall down.

The picture here inserted show how the method is practiced. The members first stand all in a row, with eyes closed. Mr. Tanaka, acting as A, then takes a deep breath, exerts the internal action of Reishi in his abdominal region and holds out his hand. At once all members of the class tumble down like surging wave. The scene presented indeed is a very remarkable one.

For beginners, however, it is advisable to practice on individuals. Let A have B stand upright with eyes closed; and then A, by inhaling deeply and charging the abdominal muscles with the internal action of Reishi, breaths strongly toward B, and the latter will fall to the ground, usually backward. Nothing in the way of other action or any suggestion is necessary. At first in such experiments the space between A and B should be about two or three feet; and as one advances in mastery of the art one may extend the space to from 20 to 30 feet, B always falling like a log. Achieving success in this way the number of those to be acted upon can be increased to 3, 5, 8 and 10, as 'A' can act upon as many as ten persons at once when he gets to be proficient in the art. Of course great care has to be taken in the practice of such an art. A has to be careful to breathe properly and to exert properly the action of Reishi in his abdominal muscles and then to breathe out strongly in the proper manner upon the person to be thrown down, who, within a few seconds, will all tumble over, as desired. It is difficult to take a picture of groups falling in this way, like the photograph of a single person falling like a tree. The picture reproduced above was taken by one of the most expert of rapid photographers.

---

[213] Sweeney has taught similar on classes since 1990s

5. Theory of the Art of Exercising the Power of Reishi on Others

From what has already been said one may gain some idea of how Reishi is utilized in the art of self-defense. Many will be disposed to ask, however, why such phenomena are possible. It is due simply to the fact when one has acquired the art of the action of Reishi in the abdominal region he can so exert it through breathing outward as to bring it to bear on the object or objects determined upon so that these objects lose all self-control. It is accomplished just in the same manner as when A causes B to go round and round in a circle. All such phenomena are caused by the power of Reishi. Of course the theory of such action is too profound for definition in words. One has to see it really to appreciate its marvellous significance and reality. Two fundamental principles, however, are involved, known as the Internal Action of Reishi and the External Action of Reishi, which one gets to apprehend fully after a course in the principles and doctrines of TAIREIDO. This is so important a part of the teaching it cannot be fully elucidated in this short introduction to the system. For full information the reader must obtain the volume entitled TAIREIDO by Mr. Morihei Tanaka.

6. Experiments Bordering on the Miraculous

At the lectures delivered by Mr. Tanaka on TAIREIDO may incidents take place which cannot be accounted for by any ordinary explanation of the application of the laws of nature, and many regard these as instances of the miraculous or supernatural element. One of the most mysterious of these facts is the art of apprehending the thought of another, mentioned above. To be able to know what is in the mind of another is truly a remarkable power. In addition to this, there are many other instances of the truly wonderful and even miraculous in connection with practicing the art of Reishi, details which cannot be given here. How this power may be utilized for the good of mankind is outlined in the succeeding chapter.

III

Application of Reishi Action to Disease

The revelation of TAIREIDO and its practical application in the Action of Reishi were not given to mankind simply for the sake of performing interesting not to say wonderful experiments in regard to the power of spirit over matter, and of mind over body; but for the amelioration and removal of human suffering[214] and the improvement and happiness of human life[215]. One of the most useful applications of the Action of Reishi is in the cure of sickness and healing of disease in every form[216]. Without use of medicine or any assistance whatever, the Action of Reishi may be used to cure sickness[217]. Disease of every kind may be removed likewise without drugs or the resort to doctors or surgery[218]. And the application of the Action of Reishi to the cure of sickness and the healing of diseases is effective independently of the faith or mental state of the patient. The practitioner can affect a cure or bring relief even if the patient does not believe in Reishi treatment, and even if there is absolute doubt or aversion to it[219].

The following is an account of the experiences of Mr. Taro Shinozaki as to sensations caused by the application of Reishi Action in surgical cases.

1. Use of Reishi in Medical Treatment

It is hardly necessary to say that the effect of the Action of Reishi in the treatment of disease differs according to the temperament, constitution and general condition of the patient as well as according to the nature of the disease to be cured. The most important condition, however, is the degree in which the power of Reishi is manifested in the practitioner. We know of a certain gentleman in Tokyo who was cured by Reishi treatment. He was 35 years of age and suffering from bronchitis as well as pleurisy; and although he had spent much time and expense in a sanatorium he was nothing bettered. He was deeply depressed on account of his illness, about the nature of which he had read in some medical book, and his future seemed hopeless.

---

[214] Usui's Hikkei states: 'amelioration of both mental and physical exercise'

[215] Usui's Hikkei mentions: 'increase of happiness in the Reiki patient and his or hers fellow patients.' It's interesting that not only is the language similar, but also that the two phrases are so close together in each document.

[216] There are similar references to how Reiki can cure – and without medicine, in various parts of Usui's Hikkei.'

[217] Similar in Usui's Hikkei says Reiki 'is a therapy that aims to cure the mind and the body.'

[218] Comments in Usui's Hikkei also say Reiki 'is not based on medicine.'

[219] Similar language again from Usui's Hikkei states Reiki 'does not therefore require an explicit consent on the part of the patient or any loyalty to the practitioner concerned. Not only that, we practitioners of the Usui Reiki Therapy do not mind however much our practices are doubted, held in contempt or rejected.'

He resorted to Buddhism for consolation in his declining health, but his pessimism continued and his condition did not improve. At this time he was also suffering from extreme nervous debility, with headache and much exhaustion. He had a bad cough and could not sleep at night. Finally in his extremity he sought the assistance of TAIREIDO, through the advice of relatives.

At first he had no faith in the Reishi treatment, and paid little or no attention to the advice given him. As he passed through the early stages of the treatment he thought there was no benefit to his health, but the practitioner could see that the patient was already beginning to show signs of improvement. During the second day of treatment the beneficial influence of Reishi was clearly revealed. There was a sudden movement of the head and hands and he could feel that the process of recovery had begun. The patient said he had been suffering extreme exhaustion from the previous day; but on the third day from the time treatment commenced he felt impelled to a sudden movement while in bed after which he felt better; then he slept two hours of unbroken comfortable sleep, to the surprise of all around him, and awoke feeling renewed and refreshed. From that time the progress of recovery was steady and rapid. Reishi was having its sure effect. It was seen that at times during the treatment the patient used to move violently and sometimes wept. Asked if he could explain why he wept he said that he did not know why, but such a feeling of relief and gratitude came over him that he could not help it. Day by day his state of exhaustion grew less. The first time of treatment he came to the practicing room in a jinrikisha, but on the third night he had his first four hours of quiet and consecutive sleep for a long time.

With the process of treatment during the fourth and fifth days his recovery continued to be most satisfactory, as he felt renewed and was gradually regaining his former strength. His shattered nerves were also beginning to feel natural again. His speech, action and general appearance had much improved, and he was calm and normal. On the sixth day it was decided to apply a special Reishi treatment, such as is used for curing illness at a distance. At first he suffered a little from the changes, the first two days showing some mental confusion; but from the third day of the new treatment exactly at the appointed hour for treatment *in absentia* he experienced a sudden, powerful influence working upon him and he fell into a condition of cheerful repose leading to some hours of the most peaceful and refreshing sleep. This treatment went on for a week, after which he was about as well as a man could be, and resumed his official duties which illness had forced him to abandon.

2. Wonderful Response to the Power of Reishi

The patient in the preceding paragraph, after some ten days of treatment at a distance, again visited the office of TAIREIDO and requested direct treatment once more, to which he submitted for about eight days. During this treatment he frequently revealed symptoms of the powerful effect of Reishi on his whole physical and mental condition; his body showed certain mysterious tremors and remarkable action. When the Reishi practitioner stood about two feet from him and applied the Action of Reishi the body of the patient indicated violent movement, with commotion within. He was then lying on a couch, face upward. When the finger of Mr. Tanaka moved nearer to him, at a distance of two or three inches from his body, the limbs of the patient moved violently; and when Mr. Tanaka retired to an adjoining room and treated him mentally at a distance the body of the patient showed violent movement. It was thus obvious to both the practitioner and the patient that the power of Reishi was something transcending space and time, the very essence on which all existence depends. On the fifth day of the renewed direct treatment the patient at a certain moment suddenly clasped his hands, as if in devotion; and afterwards explained that the action was not intentional, but the result of the Action of Reishi in his body.

A further remarkable phenomenon of the result of treatment on this patient was that on the second day of resumed direct treatment he began to have a habit of moving both hands unconsciously during the operation of Reishi, rubbing his forehead, patting his body whenever Mr. Tanaka's hand touched him. Since that time he always massaged or rubbed his body this way during Reishi treatment; and after it was over he invariably experienced a feeling of wonderful physical and mental refreshment and renewal. The fact that he rubbed his nose was due to the application of the Action of Reishi to his bronchial trouble.

3. Power of Reishi over all Ailments

After finishing his eight days of treatment under the Action of Reishi the patient above described returned and went about his usual avocations as if he had never suffered from any serious affection. Sixteen days later he returned and had four days more of direct treatment, so as to maintain progress toward immunity to return of his illness. By this time it was noticeable that he had ceased to massage himself and rub his breast and abdomen. He told Mr. Tanaka that whenever the latter touched him in the Reishi treatment he felt an indescribable sensation as of a some powerful spirit taking possession of his mind and body, penetrating to his inmost being, which thrilled him and refreshed him so that he could not restrain his emotions, sometimes to weep, but more often toward a feeling of abnormal refreshment and physical pleasure. The above is but the merest outline of some of the more interesting phases of this remarkable case of recovery from a chronic and dangerous disease.

After doing all that Mr. Tanaka could see to be necessary to the complete recovery of this patient. Mr. Tanaka brought him for examination to the head of a hospital, who carefully subjected him to the regular physical examination and diagnosis, after which he pronounced him cured of the disease and in a perfect and sound state of health, save in one place where the lung adhered to the pleura, though this in no way seemed to affect the action of the lung or to interfere with the health of the patient. The nervous debility, too, had quite disappeared. The above is a true and unvarnished account of a case that may be taken as an example of the usual result of the Action of Reishi in the treatment of illness and disease. No one but those who have suffered and thus been recovered can appreciate what Reishi means to the relief of mankind in restoring health and happiness[220].

WE believe that things necessarily come into being through the categorical imperative of *Tairei*.

IV

Reishi Independent of Time and Space

The power of Reishi to cure disease or to affect the desired result of the practitioner is quite independent of time or distance, as may be seen from the following account of the experience of a surgeon now a distinguished colonel in the Imperial army, Shogo Kasajima by name.

1. A Remarkable Patient

The patient hereafter described lived in a place far removed from the practitioner and suffered from myelitis. She was a woman named Miye

[220] Usui-sensei's Hikkei says people 'appreciate for the first time, upon being treated once, the efficacy of the Usui Reiki Therapy, and all at once, they begin to trust it'

Tsuji, 39 years old, and living in the village of Yamaguchi in Saga-ken. In the month of November, 1916 she was taken with myelitis, and womb trouble, and obliged to give up work in April of the following year. Her illness was so severe that she could do nothing but lie constantly in bed, unable to move. The upper portion of her body had much pain, while the lower portion was more or less paralyzed. She admitted to the usual medical treatment without beneficial effect. All such treatment having failed to cure her, the woman was in despair. Then she happened to read a brief account of the benefits of TAIREIDO in a magazine, and she asked our office to treat her. As she could not move to us she was content to have treatment at a distance. This began on August 4, 1917 and was to continue for a week. The treatment proper did not, however, begin until August 10, as we had in the meantime to give her proper directions. Through a mistake on her part, however, she thought the treatment was to begin on August 7, and consequently remained quietly in expectation of it and the resulting benefit. But for three days she felt no relief at all. On the 10th as she was lying in bed still hoping for some benefit, she learned that the treatment did not actually begin until that day. About eight o'clock that evening and half-past eight she fell into a deep sleep, just at the time when the treatment was being applied a long distance away - All of the sudden the woman felt aroused from sleep as if awakened by someone; and she asked the attendant what time it was. He said it was just half-past eight. She requested her nurse to withdraw; and then tried to sit up in the bed, removing her upper garment and facing the south, as if being treated by a physician actually in the room. After thus waiting a few minutes she felt the lower part of her body begin to experience tremors and then to move more violently, and she thus trembled as if the life would tremble out of her, as she said. At first the result was a feeling of something grotesque and fearsome; but her brain became quite clear and she felt something like electricity shooting through her fingers, and ran like pins and needles all over her body. In the place she felt as if an insect had stung her. Then came a queer pain in her loins, and she felt unable to sit up for the required half hour, the period appointed for her treatment. This pain was at the beginning of the treatment; but no sooner had the latter begun than the pain vanished and she felt no further discomfort. For the thirty-minutes of Reishi treatment the woman was absolutely comfortable, save for the strange feeling resulting from the application of the Action of Reishi.

The second period of treatment was to be from 8:30 to 9 p.m. on the following day; but the nurse had forgotten to inform her of this; and consequently at 8 o'clock when she was expecting to experience the effect of the treatment she felt nothing unusual, and asked the attendant what time it was. Then at 8:40 she suddenly felt an unusual communion in her body and asked the nurse again what time it was, and was told it was forty minutes past eight. During the period of treatment on this evening the woman experienced exactly the same feelings as on the previous evening under treatment; and on the third evening the same feelings and experiences were likewise repeated. On the evening of the 13th, however, she felt rather an unusual movement that caused her to clasp her hands in wonder. Her fingers moved and were beyond her control. They moved of themselves. It was impossible for her to remain sitting in bed under such emotion and movement and so she had to lie down, simply feeling that she was being treated by the Action of Reishi, as agreed upon. Her hands remained clasped and her fingers continued to move convulsively as before. She unclasped them again, and they began to move of themselves, the motion growing stronger and stronger, and the space of their movement being over one foot.

Thus her experience went on to the 24th of the month, the treatment proceeding over the hundreds of miles between Tokyo and Saga, and then the woman wrote that she had wonderful experience and felt much better already. She could now get out of bed and walk with the assistance of a cane, remaining up from two to three hours at a time. Under the application of the Action of Reishi this woman continued to recover, the pain departed and her natural complexion returned; and after five weeks of treatment she considered herself as well as ever, only she had still to be careful as to diet. She wrote to the office of TAIREIDO a letter couched in the most courteous terms and filled with gratitude for the benefits our treatment had bestowed upon her.

2. Fifteen Years of Illness

The following is an accurate description of a case of gout from which Mr. Zenji Tanno, aged 60, had suffered for over 15 years. Mr. Tano lives at Terauchi in Fukushima ken, and was very ill with the above mentioned ailment. He entered the Tokyo University Hospital for the usual treatment, one of the most famous hospitals of the empire, but without benefit; and he tried other good hospitals, with the same unsatisfactory result. His ailment was in no way made better. Abandoning all medical treatment as hopeless he went to various mineral springs to take hot baths; and this he did for years, only realizing that with time he was getting worse instead of better. It was an obstinate disease that gave him much pain and constant discomfort, especially during changes of season, and changeable weather. His physical condition was gradually weakening and the flesh of the limbs growing flabby. He at last heard of our Reishi treatment and decided to submit to it from a distance. After two weeks he completely cured and able to go about his work as if he had never been ill.

We have on record another case of a man who had suffered from cancer of the stomach and who was cured of the dread disease by treatment by Reishi for only 13 weeks. This patient, Mr. Choernon Sosaki, lives just in front of Kogota station at Oudagori in Miyagi ken. At the age of fifty he found himself suffering from cancer of the stomach, and for years spent much under the treatment of various physicians, some of them great experts, but instead of being cured he felt the disease gradually growing worse, eating out his life. The case is worth special consideration since cancer is considered incurable. It certainly is incurable by ordinary medical treatment. Yet it responds to Reishi without difficulty.

In his great disappointment and distress Mr. Sosaki wrote to the office of TAIREIDO asking for long-distance treatment. This was on the 12th of August, 1918. At the time he was in great torment and unable to eat anything. His stomach was swollen and pain was constant, with great irregularity of the system. He had constipation and dysentery alternately. His appearance was emaciated and anemic, and he was fast losing weight. He could not walk to his room. But after thirteen weeks of treatment from the action of Reishi he was perfectly cured, and we have a courteous letter from him gladly acknowledging his marvellous recovery under our treatment.

3. Other Cases of Marvellous Recovery

Some time ago a medical student named Mr. Kenichiro Shimada came to the office of TAIREIDO suffering from a grave nervous ailment. This gentleman was a student at the Tohoku Imperial University Medical College at Sendai, and lives at 166 Kamisugiyama-dori, Kitagoban-cho, in that city. Being obliged by illness to give up study Mr. Shimada appealed to us for treatment. It was a very troublesome case of nervous exhaustion. He could not use his head at all, and was irritable, suffering from insomnia as well. He had severe indigestion and general inactivity of the system. As his university examination was coming on he felt rather depressed and hopeless; and as a last resort he asked for Reishi treatment. After only one week of application of Reishi at a distance he was quite recovered and in normal health, and after another week he was better than ever. In this case there was a very remarkable tremor of the body during treatment.

There is another case where we have the thanks of a doctor for complete recovery after treatment by the application of the Action of Reishi. Dr. Tani is a physician living in Wakayagi, Kurihara-gori in Miyagi ken. One day, he came to the office of TAIREIDO with his wife and grandson. Without giving any indication as to the ailment of his wife he simply asked us to examine her. It was soon discovered that there was a growth about four inches in diameter near the womb, the tumor being filled with liquid. The doctor was obviously surprised at our rapid and accurate diagnosis of the trouble. He then asked us if we could undertake to treat the woman, and said his grandchild also needed treatment.

The history of the case is interesting, in view of the cure obtained. This woman was 73 years old and suffered from phthisis for some twenty years. She also had asthma and heart trouble, having been treated by physicians for many years, without receiving benefit. After three weeks treatment by our office she is almost cured, having now only a little cough at times. Soon she will be as well as ever.

Kumiji, her granddaughter, is 23 years old, and had long suffered from stomach and bowel disease, receiving no benefit from medical treatment. She could eat little or nothing and had obstruction in the intestines. Her only relief from pain was from morphine injections. She had to be fed artificially in order to prolong life. The she came under our Reishi treatment at a distance. Within ten days the vomiting stopped and she could take food, the pain in the stomach gradually stopping. The case in fact responded to the Action of Reishi and will soon be completely cured, to the great joy of the woman.

The cases above mentioned are only those where cure from ordinary medical treatment was manifestly impossible. Cases of recovery from ordinary illness through Reishi treatment are so numerous and common that we forbear to cite any of them; but the above instances of complete recovery from apparently incurable maladies under the application of the Action of Reishi are so remarkable and extraordinary, they are to be marvellous if not miraculous. They prove the effective power of Reishi under all circumstances; and yet there is no real wonder about it, for the power that caused all things to exist must be able to affect all good for mankind when properly used. If any desire further information as to cases cured and treatment offered they may correspond with the TAIREIDO Association.

TAIREIDO has its system of teaching the fundamental principles of the Art of applying the Action of Reishi for all purposes of improving human life[221] and existence. Instruction may be either by attending the classes in our

---

[221] Usui's Hikkei says almost identically, 'improving mankind's enjoyment of human life'

office or by correspondence and reading our literature. Any on may easily acquire the art by applying to us and following our directions: We fit the pupil thoroughly for the practice of such arts as Reishi, including the art of apprehending what is in the mind of others, of thought transmission to others, of apprehending physical condition, spirit photography, prophecy, and many other occult arts[222] of which the human mind and body are capable under due instruction from experts.

For fuller information as to the whole system of TAIREIDO and all it does for mankind, one should read the volume entitled TAIREIDO, A New Revelation for the elimination of diseases and the improvement of life[223]*, by Morihei Tanaka, founder of TAIREIDO, published by our Association and to be had by applying to our office in Tokyo*[224]*. This volume gives a full statement in detail of the secrets of Art of Reishi.*

WE believe that all the things in the world are rational; and that this rationality has proceeded from the divine will of *Tairei*.

---

[222] Subjects Tanaka supports are also in the Theosophy movement that was big news globally in late 1800s and early 1900s. Since late 1990s Sweeney taught Theosophy may be Reiki's roots, and suggested his students study works by Mdm Blavatski, CW Leadbeater, A Besant and A Bailey. Historians can decide if Tanaka, being a learned and well-read man, had an understanding of Theosophy from Theosophists who visited Japan in that era?

[223] This book includes the volume suggested here to be read.

[224] These writings pre-date Usui-sensei. If writings of Tanaka could be read by applying to his office in Tokyo; and if the writings were public knowledge (they were actually quite famous, being in Japanese newspapers); and if Usui-sensei was a learned man (which he was) and read widely; it is highly likely Usui-sensei who also lived in Tokyo had read about Tanaka.

TAIREIDO[225]

TAIREIDO, or the Great-Spirit-Way, is a new doctrine of life recently systematized and taught by a Japanese thinker named Morihei Tanaka of Tokyo. The idea that if one has a proper conception of the universe and is able to grasp the force and meaning of cosmic thought and cosmic processes he will have control over nature and self, even to the extent of eliminating evil and disease[226]. Tanaka's idea is to recognise man's knowledge of science, philosophy and religion and give a newer and truer interpretation to human life and experience. His system of thought as derived from physical research, he calls Science of Reishi, the practical application of which he calls the Art of Reishi.

According to his system the external world is a reality; and so is the conscious, thinking subject, man. The phenomenal world which man recognizes is Reishi; but behind this lays the ultimate reality, called Tairei, or Great-Spirit, which exists beyond the region of experience. The whole universe is a living system of cosmic life; and everything in it is but a manifestation of the cosmic life. The universe, however, is not infinite but finite.

Mind and matter are but manifestations of the Reishi, or essence of the universe. The nature of this dynamic principle is productive and creative force by virtue of which all things, visible and invisible, come into being according to laws of rhythm. The force of the cosmic spirit, or Reishi, is felt everywhere, as mind and matter, coming either out of an original spring whence all things rise and toward which all things ultimately return. Mind and matter, though apparently different, are one and the same manifestation of *Reishi*, the life of the universe. Whether this life is finite or not depends on whether the universe is finite; for this force is the life of the universe.

Tairei, or Great Spirit, is the ultimate reality the real nature of which emanates in various forms as phenomena, the manifestation being possible only through the creative force of *Reishi*, or Spirit-force - The Tairei is absolute and infinite; yet it gives rise to *Reishi*, or Spirit-force, which is the cosmic force of creation. In the Tanaka system of thought the universe

[225] This is an article published in the Japan Magazine in 1917 – see footnote at end of this article.

[226] These words are loosely connected to the Hikkei of Usui which says, 'Any being who has received the gift of belonging to the Universe is equipped with this therapy's spiritual power'

simply means the phenomenal world of experience; and so the universe can be no more infinite than the world of phenomena. The universe is none the less a living organism implying intelligence in origin and process, else man could perceive nothing spiritual in it.

Man's knowledge is limited to relations of time and space, apart from which, though both be merely subjective, he can have no knowledge whatever. The Reality that is beyond the limits of time and space man can have no knowledge of. Only one thing can be predicated of Reality: it is an emanation through the creative force of *Reishi*, or Spirit-power; and is this manifested. The essence of *Reishi* is neither spiritual nor physical but the force that brings all things out of Reality. The great Reality itself may be called Tairei, or Great Spirit; but when regarded from the point of view of activity or manifestation it must be called *Reishi*, or Spirit-force. Mind and matter are products of *Reishi*, which in turn is the product of Tairei. It is by reason of the omnipresent nature of Tairei manifesting itself constantly in Reishi that we behold an endless succession of events in this world. Both Tairei and Reishi are everywhere and at all times present; but as man is unable to distinguish strictly between inorganic and organic being, he is unable to distinguish between Tairei and *Reishi* in actual existence. If it is possible to posit a world where no event whatever takes place, it is also possible to think of Tairei existing alone there by reason of its nature with no relation to anything else. But once this Reality allows force to issue from it, things material or spiritual must of necessity be produced.

The idea of Nirvana, or non-being, taught in Buddhism is a slight approach to the conception of Tairei, but the idea of *Reishi*, which can exist over and above the universe itself, is quite new. As an illustration of the relation between Reality and its Manifestation we may take the well-known example of water and waves. If we look upon water as *Reishi*, Tairei, or Reality may be looked upon as the universe which contains both water and waves. Thus the great Reality is permanent, while the manifestation thereof may be transient and finite, giving rise to the phenomenal world of our experience. Nothing arising out of the law of the conservation of energy or the indestructibility of matter can change these facts. The inconstancy of the actual world is due to finiteness of *Reishi*, proceeding from the infinite Reality, or Tairei.

The atomic theory of matter bears witness to the truth of the spiritual force issuing from Reality underlying all matter. The relation of atoms is according to laws of rhythm fixed by the force of *Reishi*. Anything produced by Reishi according to the laws of rhythm must be regarded as a living or organic system. The world is a living organism; and is filled with living organized bodies or communities. Thus the activity of the *Reishi*, or Cosmic Spirit-force, is both actual, or kinetic; and also potential; a distinction that must be constantly borne in mind.

It is, therefore, a mistake to suppose that the activity of *Reishi* is a mystery beyond the mind of man. Even in physical science man learns something of the laws of its working. Not only so, but by following the proper method man may become possessed of the *Reishi*, or Spirit-force of the Great Reality, Tairei. Once in possession of the Power man can do things impossible to physics and physiology. He can control his mental and physical condition perfectly, even to the extent of lifting above the laws of gravitation, and get rid of physical disease. By gaining the force of *Reishi* man can also cure the disease of his fellow men. The power of radium, which is so much discussed today, is nothing compared with the power of *Reishi*, and the cosmic forced by which all things stand. It is not a mystery beyond the mind of man, but a possession awaiting his acceptance. It comes to man from personal contact and communion with Tairei, or the Great Reality. By possession of the force issuing from the Great Reality man is freed from the limitations of human nature, and transcends he limits of both time and space. He can even see the unbroken past and determine the continuous future. He can reclaim the good that the ignorance of man has discarded, and bring the masses of the people to intelligence and justice.

How one can enjoy possession of this good for himself and his fellow Men is the instruction that Mr. Tanaka undertakes to give in his doctrine of the laws of *Reishi*, wherein the theoretical sides are fully treated, representing a system of human salvation as this teacher by his study of science, religion and philosophy conceives it. He believes that by fixing man's faith in the ultimate Reality and acquiring the power by which the ultimate Reality works, man can achieve the ideals of his spirit as guided by Spirit of the Universe. Thus man can reach a perfect system of ethics, morality and progress.

To many the new teaching will not seem so new, especially to Christians, who call the ultimate Reality God the Father, the *Reishi*, or Spirit-force, the Holy Spirit, and the manifestation in time, the Christ, or Incarnation of God. Christians have long believed, even if they have not always practiced it, that the potential power of the Absolute God was at their disposal through the Holy Spirit, even to the extent of healing moral and physical disease. Various attempts have been made to improve on the Christian idea of such possibility, or to make up for the Church's neglect of it, among which may be mentioned Christian Science, Faith Healing and many other cults or creeds. Mr. Tanaka's way will probably appear to some as but one more attempt in the same direction. It matters nothing, of course, by what names we call things, so long as the meaning and the application are the same. And the ideas represented in Mr. Tanaka's system are certainly similar to those propounded in Christian doctrine. There is an important aspect of the Tanaka system, however, which truth cannot afford to ignore. He may have found some rational and practical way of acquiring the Spirit-force of the universe for which man has always longed. Reason would certainly dictate that there should be some way of acquiring such power by those fitted to use it in an altruistic and intelligent manner, just as man has acquired means of utilizing electric power. Of course it is futile to argue that electric power is neither moral nor immoral, but mere force the morality of which depends on the user. The force of *Reishi*, as outlined by Mr. Tanaka, is doubtless the same. In fact all the good things that Heaven has bestowed on man depend on his intelligent use for their moral effect. Even the best things can be prostituted to base purposes. Therefore it is no argument against Mr. Tanaka's doctrine that God would not be likely to delegate such power to imperfect mortals on this earth. Great power is already delegated to man, which he can use for good or ill, as he, by virtue of his moral character, determines. Those who wish to know more of Mr. Tanaka's teaching and methods may do so by communicating with the Editor of the Japan Magazine, 6 Itchome Uchisaiwai-ch, Kojimachi-ku, Tokyo.

The Japan Magazine, August, 1917[227].

WE believe that the nature of a community, independent of all determinations, temporal and spatial, is the most real and perfect.

---

[227] The Japan Magazine published this account of Tanaka's work in 1917, and asked readers who wished to know more to contact their office in Tokyo. As Usui-sensei lived in Tokyo and was well-read, it is highly likely he read this article; or at least that the article was known to him.

TAIREIDO

[228]Some time ago an article appeared in the pages of the Japan Magazine dealing with the new system of thought revealed to me by divine providence, and since then I have had so many requests for further light on the subject that I venture now to offer a few remarks in relation thereto, though no adequate conception of a system of thought that involves the fundamental essence of life and all things, can be given in a short magazine article. To receive appreciable benefit application should be made for literature dealing with this subject, and if possible to me personally.

Speaking briefly I may say that the doctrine and teaching of TAIREIDO embrace the entire nature of TAIREI, the Supreme Spirit, or fundamental essence of all things, and lead the human mind to complete Truth, as well as to that perfection of development and life for which man was created.

The system of TAIREIDO embraces and yet transcends all Religion, Philosophy, Science and Ethics. Indeed it is a system of thought that exhausts the Truth of the universe, and defies the real meaning and significance of human life.

The Supreme object of TAIREIDO is to unify human thought so as to bring mankind everywhere and therefore peace to the world. TAIREIDO gives perfect health of both mind and body to man. It reveals the fundamental principles of human society and the basis of true national life for all mankind. TAIREIDO develops and perfects the intellectual faculties of man and reconstructs human civilization on an eternal foundation.

Would that I could make my voice heard with this message to the entire world! As one surveys the world today it is clear that the greater portion of mankind has lost the real significance of existence and fails to recognise the true value of human life. There is much physical and intellectual toil and yet no finding of the path that leads to true manhood and womanhood. Mankind lacks a true centre of thought, and has no conception of the absolute nature of things and therefore no reverence for truth and divine reality. The wandering mind of man is thus at sea as to any sure dependence, and life for most people is unceasing bewilderment. No one can truly affirm today that the trend of human thought is in line with truth. In spite of the universal and eager haste for satisfaction of human intelligence there is no real reflection,

---

[228] The following is an article by Tanaka that was published in The Japan Magazine in 1918. It is largely a copy of his work published earlier in this book, with adjustments to language and inclusion/exclusion of paragraphs.

no perception of introspection. If this process continues, human society may only descend to disintegration and ruin. The war in Europe is only a trifle compared with what awaits mankind ignorant of its true destiny. Even without such cataclysms humanity will come to ruin simply for want of capacity for introspection. The war has its appointed end, but the fatal lack of introspection goes on.

It is man's custom to talk of great progress and to boast of modern enlightenment; but it is quite evident that human society has not as yet reached a stage beyond mere mass and inorganic substance. To thrill this human mass with real life, and penetrate it with absolute thought is the only hopes of being relived of the present darkness and inertia and led along the pathway of light and life. As capacity for introspection develops, and new light begins to dawn, the way of life becomes clear. It is from introspection that all phenomena of the world take rise. It is through introspection alone that the human mind can perceive the true light and follow the true way.

Hitherto mankind has been looking in vain to religions like Buddhism and Christianity for the way of light. These religions still dominate the mind of large sections of the human race. But man has now reached a stage where such religions can do little to lead him toward his true goal of human existence, the kingdom of introspection which is man's kingdom of Heaven. The more man trusts to these vanities today the more hopelessly bewildered will he find himself and the darker will grow his hope. The present is indeed a time of real crisis for humanity. Unless we realize our mental paralysis and come to the true source of thought and life the future offers no light.

One of the most impressive facts of the last hundred years has been the marvellous progress of physical science. So rapid and far-reaching has been the increase of knowledge and invention that if our ancestors should suddenly return to the earth they would faint from sheer amazement. A century ago not even the most sanguine of prophets would have dared to predict such progress as modern civilization has attained. Yet no one that has observed the real condition of human life will deny that its improvement has not kept peace with its material prosperity. Indeed, it is open to grave doubt whether, side by side with this material advancement, man has shown any adequate sign of the most advanced nations. While our ancestors would probably be astonished at the outward progress of their posterity, they would undoubtedly be correspondingly shocked at our lack of mental and moral development.

The civilization of our time is essentially nothing more than a mere materialization and mechanization of humanity. As the scientist resolves all substances into atoms or molecules, so any accurate analysis of mankind today reveals only a mass of mediocrity, as alike as the atoms of matter, without a mind to master the body that clothes them. What better than a machine is the average person we know! Humanity seems to have lost all consciousness of its inherent greatness; man no longer exhibits the enduring and substantial character of his ancestors. These are, of course, some slight indications of humanity awakening to a sense of what has been lost or never attained; there are signs of a desire to recover or reach man's natural greatness, and to escape from complexity and confusion of our soulless and mechanical civilization. But there is yet very little progress in the realization of man's dawning desire.

While amply aware of the progress of our material civilization, we nevertheless have no real desire to be enmeshed in its coils, or crushed in its machinery. We duly recognise the degree of thought attained by our forebears, but yet we cannot deny its great imperfection. What man most wants is spiritual civilization as far transcending the present material civilization as now the latter does the former. The thought of today, on which man's real progress depends, should transcend the civilization of our time as well as transcend the thought of the past. Only as man approaches this spiritual civilization will he attain unto the divine state that transcends all mind and matter, the culture of the real superman.

No study of the past or present, however profound, can bring any peace or satisfaction to the mind and soul of man, no matter how much he may value them. While material advancement goes on, mental and spiritual progress lags behind, and man is unable to face the new duties that constantly arise. Into this gulf between mind and matter, between material civilization and mental retardation, comes the new revelation to man, known as TAIREIDO, the essence and thought of all created things as well as of things uncreated, the only reality that transcends matter and mind, and yet the foundation of all mental and material development. TAIREIDO is not the product but the producer of thought and life. Because of its absence from materialistic civilization of today the world is threatened with human retrogression.

The Art of Reishi, which is the system by which TAIREIDO manifests its power in human life, imparts to man the divine capacity to reach his full consummation of mind and body. Thereby man attains to spiritual supremacy over matter, especially over the substance of which he is composed. Man is more than physical raiment that encloses him. TAIREIDO enable man to transcend mind and matter, to rise above the confusion of philosophy, science and religion.

Having devoted my life to this truth I can vouch for its reality and importance, as can the thousands who have also tested it and found it true. Therefore with the most absolute assurance I proclaim to the world the doctrine of TAIREIDO, knowing that only through acquirement of this truth can mankind attain unto transcendent thought, and the life that is its fruit.

The Japan Magazine, December, 1918

TAIREIDO

We have received a new volume entitled TAIREIDO explaining a unique system of thought and life revealed to the author Mr. Morihei Tanaka. This gentleman has for some time been attracting wide attention in Japan and the Far East as the Expounder of Taireido, which now has quite a large number of disciples[229]. The new system of thought is certainly one of the most remarkable guesses at the Riddle of the Universe that we have come across in recent years. To Mr. Tanaka and his followers, however, it is no guess but a revelation of the fundamental truths of existence. It would, of course, be quite impossible in the space at our disposal to give any adequate account of this wonderful system of thought as laid down in the volume under review. Mr. Tanaka has contributed various articles to our pages[230] with reference to the subject, and his remarks have elicited wide interest, judging by the number of inquiries received. It will be sufficient at this time merely to say that the founder of TAIREIDO claims to have had revealed to him, after a long period of bodily discipline, the secret of all existence. It was a revelation from the Great Spirit who is the author of all things. From this experience the author of Taireido saw that the essence of things is neither material nor spiritual but a fusion of these; and that man, the highest product of this fusion, has within himself the power of the Spirit to regulate his body, his soul, as well as human society and civilization in harmony with the law of the universe, without which evil must prevail. Once man has acquired the secret of this inherent power, by instruction in Taireido, he can

---

[229] Because Usui-sensei lived in Tokyo, and was an intelligent and widely read man, he most likely read this and the previous two articles published in The Japan Magazine, especially as Taireido and Reishi had 'quite a large number of disciples'.

[230] The Japan Magazine states Tanaka previously had published 'various articles' in their magazine, not only the one article by him presented in this book.

regulate his physical, mental and moral functions in accordance with the laws of the universe, or in harmony with TRUTH, as Mr. Tanaka says; so that all irregularity and disease are eliminated from mankind. Man can wield this divine power both for himself and for others. By the same power all creation has been produced; and by this power man can bring his life into unity with creation. The power can be exercised everywhere at all times, unlimited by distance or circumstance. The author claims that this new system of thought and life supersedes all the spiritual and intellectual knowledge so far acquired by mankind. Needless to say such teaching has created no small interest in Japan, where Mr. Tanaka has attracted much attention during the past few years; and considerable numbers of people are not only displaying keen interest in it but are placing themselves under the instruction of the author of Taireido[231], including all classes from the highest to the lowest[232]. Some quite wonderful results of the effect on individuals have been recorded, and the book itself gives numerous examples, as well as explaining lucidly the general principles of the system. This volume, thus compiled out of the author's marvellous experience, is intended for students of Taireido living too far from the author to come personally under his instruction. Particulars as to the volume, or as to Taireido, itself, may be had by applying to the office of the Japan Magazine[233].

[*Review in the Japan Magazine.*]

---

[231] Confirmation from The Japan Magazine that, 'considerable numbers' of people were interested in and were studying Tanaka's system of Taireido and Reishi. Once again, it seems highly unlikely that Usui-sensei did not at least know of Tanaka's work.

[232] Usui's Hikkei mentions similar, that those who do Reiki are from 'eminent scholars, both male and female, to the illiterate.'

[233] Yet again, before Usui sensei taught Reiki in Tokyo, this provides sound evidence that Tanaka's writings on healing with Taireido and Reishi were available openly to the public, this time courtesy of The Japan Society's Tokyo office near where Usui-sensei lived.

大正九年七月十日印刷
大正九年七月十五日發行

編輯兼發行者　伊藤延次
東京市京橋區銀座四丁目一番地
印刷者　村岡徹三
東京市京橋區銀座四丁目一番地
印刷所　ジヤパン・マガジーン印刷所
東京市麹町區一番町四十二番地
發行所　太靈道本院

[END]

Appendix 1

How Usui's writings were discovered by guidance!

This copy of an article was originally published about 11 years ago before Shortt discovered this book by Tanaka. It is re-printed here because Sweeney's guided discovery of Usui's writings in 1998 seems relevant to the discovery of the writings in this book.

1998 saw a startling discovery that changed the Reiki world. Dr Allan Sweeney was the first Reiki sensei from outside Japan to be invited to lecture at the inaugural gathering of Japanese Reiki Masters in Tokyo, and at the same time be given Dr Usui's original writings, which changed Reiki consciousness. (Similarly this book by Tanaka could open the consciousness of the Reiki world.)

Allan has been guided by Dr Usui since he appeared to him in 1995, saying in no uncertain terms he was worthy enough to teach Reiki. William Rand watched Allan's hands rise high in the air, and said he knew something special had happened. Many students have now seen Usui on Allan's courses - even on his face. Often, Usui's guidance taught Allan different knowledge that was later shown to be Usui teaching.

In early 1998 Akiko Ono, one of Allan's London students, was about to visit Japan. Allan asked her to find answers to 40 questions on Reiki's uncertain history. She didn't know how, so Allan said she'd be guided – but didn't realize guidance would come from him on 3 different occasions.

In Japan, Akiko could not find answers. But she remembered Allan said she'd be guided, and felt guided to her phone directory. As she flicked through the pages, she said she became aware of a hand taking hers. (She was convinced it was Allan's left hand.) The hand guided her to a phone number on a certain page. Akiko was surprised. It was the Chief Student of the 6th President of Dr Usui's society, Hiroshi Doi! He was hardly ever at home, but was there for just half an hour!

Japanese social rules say you cannot just phone for an appointment - you must first know a name and address; and one of their friends who checks if they wish to meet; then receive a written invitation. However, Hiroshi Doi liked her story of being guided, invited her to dinner, and to a lecture about the History of Reiki as taught by Dr Usui's own Society.

At the meeting Akiko saw Allan appear like a guide next to Doi. Doi then gave her many writings such as a photocopy draft of Doi's Reiki book, and Usui's 'Reiki Ideals' in his own hand-writing

One of Allan's questions for Akiko was of the mountain where Usui discovered Reiki. Doi told Akiko of a spot on Mt Kurama connected to Dr Usui and his attunements, where his Society still attunes people today. The path up Mt Kurama is steep. As Akiko climbed up, breathless, she came to steep steps, and thought that she'd have to rest. But a figure appeared. She thought, 'Is that you, Allan!' This was the third occasion she was guided by Allan. The figure strode away, not up the steep steps, but through woods. Akiko thought, 'If Allan is going that way, I had better follow him!' It was a short cut, leading direct to the spot where Dr Usui discovered Reiki.

Soon after, Doi-sensei posted a copy of Dr Usui's writings to England, and invited Allan to Japan to lecture to the first gathering of Japanese Reiki Masters. Allan was surprised to learn mystical guidance from Usui-sensei about his techniques was actually the reality of true Usui teachings.

Japanese etiquette says information should be slowly released. Allan honored this custom, so did not publish Usui's original writings. However, other persons soon published the same material... Perhaps the discovery of this original book by Tanaka, exactly 11 years after Allan discovered Usui's original writings, is another mystical opportunity to open the consciousness of all concerned.

Appendix 2

Dr Usui's Explanation of Reiki Therapy - Hikkei

This document is included as it is an original translation of Dr Usui's writings, and an introduction by Japanese masters, as given to Allan Sweeney and translated by the speechwriter/translator to the Japanese ambassador in London.

The speechwriter and Sweeney agreed that:

> *"The following document is in original 1920s language and portrays an overview of many of Dr Usui's healing and spiritual philosophies together with an insight that he was an intelligent, articulate, educated, knowledgeable man. He knew his Reiki subject in depth, and was a humble but strong character, not afraid to speak his mind if he understood a truth."*

It is interesting to note, especially when there appears to be so much confusion about how Reiki should be taught, that the teachings of Dr Usui and Mrs Takata were very, very different.

In particular note that Dr Usui did not just place hands on and rely on the intelligent nature of Reiki to do the work. He taught many techniques, and talked many times about the ability to cure in different ways. And he had extra levels of teachings only available to an inner circle.

Please note:

> *1. Japanese personal names are notoriously difficult so the translator therefore makes an educated guess with a question mark.*
>
> *2. The first 5 paragraphs are written in late 1990s Japanese, as a modern-day introduction to Dr Usui's public explanation of Usui Reiki Therapy.*
>
> *3. The subsequent explanation of Reiki Therapy and answers to questions are in the first person and is either Dr Usui's own writing, or by someone who wrote down his words.*

Attention: Mr. Allan Sweeney, Reiki International

From: [234]

Re: "Explanation of Reiki Therapy"

Date: 19th January 1999[235]

It is possible to get an impression of Dr Mikao Usui that has been traditionally handed down to us, but now a sharper image has been gradually emerging.

We have received articles contributed by Members of this Association who have been delighted to have the opportunity to get closer to the founder of this method of healing, whereas hitherto they had had only vague impressions of the master.

We also received enquiries asking whether only those persons particularly involved in the teaching handed down could familiarize themselves with the records pertaining to Dr Usui's public explanation of the Usui Reiki Therapy.

Therefore, with this special issue, we have decided to make public for the benefit for the Members of this Association the "Explanation of Reiki Therapy" which forms a part of the precious materials published by Dr [?] Yunosuke[236] Yanagihara. He is the direct inheritor of the Usui Reiki Therapy, and his collection is kept by the Human & Trust Research Institute.

---

[234] The translator of Dr Usui's document, who prefers to remain anonymous, was a respected speechwriter for London's Japanese ambassador, and understood classical 1920s Japanese. (Because the Japanese language has evolved so rapidly within the past 100 years, most modern-day people in Japan cannot understand 1920s Japanese language.) It took much time and a series of co-incidences via the Japanese Embassy to find a gifted translator who could deeply understand the now near-obsolete style of handwriting used by Dr Usui.

[235] In 1998/9, I felt the time was not right for its release. The Japanese tradition is for the slow release of information and I wished to honour this. It felt important to me that both the timing and the method of release should be the 'correct' one.

[236] According to the translator, Japanese first names are extremely difficult to translate.

As practitioners of Reiki Therapy in this age, we hope that our Members, by getting to know through this text how Dr Usui in his day approached Reiki and proclaimed it to the world, will be able to study the origins of Reiki, and together, without forgetting any of the essentials, appreciate the principles of Reiki even further.

Explanation of Reiki Therapy

By the founder, Dr Mikao Usui

From ancient times, each household has discovered its own secret cures[237], and passed them on only through their children and their grandchildren. In doing so, a family aimed to ensure its stable survival into later ages. It regarded this therapeutic knowledge as something handed down from previous centuries, not to be disclosed to people outside the family. In an age, however, when as present, the basis of human happiness is co-existence and co-prosperity, requiring social advance, this secretive approach to medicine is totally unacceptable[238].

The Usui Reiki Therapy is something no one before has discovered[239], and bears comparison with no other treatment in the world[240]. On this understanding, we make known the Reiki Therapy for the benefit of the public in the hope that many people will receive Heaven's blessing, ensuring the unity of body and soul[241], thereby enjoying natural welfare. From its origins, the Usui Reiki Therapy has been an innovative spiritual therapy[242] based on universal spiritual powers[243]. First of all, therefore, it makes

---

[237] Similarly, one of Dr Usui's Reiki objectives was to cure all ills with different 'secret' techniques.

[238] By analogy, Dr Usui wished the Reiki therapy not to be secret, but to be openly available to all.

[239] This statement by Dr Usui contradicts many books that say Reiki was 're-discovered'.

[240] Some books suggest that Reiki originated in Tibet. In Dr Usui's mind, Reiki is unique, and not to be compared with any treatment from any other country.

[241] Wholeness of being, curing and unifying body, mind, and soul is a recurring theme for Dr Usui.

[242] This is an acknowledgment that spiritual powers help Reiki, not just one spiritual force.

[243] Explaining that the origins of Reiki are a unique spiritual innovation.

persons healthy[244], and at the same time improves their mind[245], thereby improving mankind's enjoyment of human life[246].

This is why I[247] take it upon myself to proclaim the Usui Reiki Therapy to my fellow creatures who require some relief from illnesses that are giving them pain both internally and externally[248].

Question: What is the nature of the Usui Reiki Therapy?

Answer: I absorbed the last teachings graciously handed down by the late Emperor Meiji [1868~1912], refining my own doctrine[249]. In aiming for the amelioration of both mental and physical exercise and progress upon a righteous way of life, it is first necessary to cure the spirit[250], and secondly to cure the physical body[251]. If the spirit is healthy, following the path of truth, the body will become healthy of itself[252].

In this way, it is possible to enjoy a life which brings together the soul and the body and which gives pleasure in the peaceful union of the soul and the body[253]. This attitude also leads to the cure of other patients[254]. This very

---

244 The initial goal of Reiki is to improve health, which in turn helps mankind improve other levels.

245 Mental healing is part of Reiki.

246 Enjoyment of life is a main goal. See below.

247 In the first person, so this is either Dr Usui's handwriting or a direct transcription of his words.

248 Reiki heals all inner and outer aspects of a human being.

249 Dr Usui uses the Five Ideals and Waka poetry of the Meiji Emperor to enhance a righteous way of life in his students.

250 This corresponds to the common Western Reiki 1 - spiritual rei energy is used to heal a student's soul and spirit.

251 This is taught on many Western Reiki 2 classes - using the first symbol to help physical problems.

252 A 'classic' spiritual healing philosophy, showing Dr Usui as a knowledgeable healer who understands spiritual rei healing has eventual automatic knock-on effects for physical healing.

253 Classic Reiki 1 & 2 offering the energy options to heal first the soul and then the body.

254 The first attitude is to self-heal, but others can then be cured.

increase of happiness in the Reiki patient and his or hers fellow patients is the mission of Usui Reiki Therapy[255].

Q: Is not the Usui Reiki Therapy just another name for saiminjutsu (a form of hypnotism), kiaijutsu (another form of hypnotism), faith healing, or other methods of healing[256]?

A: On no account is the Usui Reiki Therapy practically the same as the techniques you have mentioned. It is a therapy that aims to cure the mind and the body, whereby I have been inspired by esoteric beliefs over a long period of rigorous study and arduous training[257].

Q: In that case, is it a spiritualistic therapy?

A: The Usui Reiki Therapy may certainly be termed a spiritualistic method of curing[258], but many of the aspects of the therapy may be called material therapy[259]. The practitioner radiates a spirit and light from every part of his or her body[260]. This spirit and light are manifested mostly in the eyes, the mouth and the hands. For this reason, the practitioner will carefully study the diseased part of the body for two or three minutes[261], breathe back on the patient[262], or massage the patient with the hands[263]. By these means, inflammation will recede from the sites of tooth-ache, abdominal pain, gastro-enteritis, neurological pain, mastitis, scars, burns,

---

[255] If someone is healed spiritually, in the soul, physically and mentally, that person will be happy! Therefore Dr Usui's first mission statement is to increase happiness.

[256] No different to today, when Reiki practitioners and masters have to defend about what Reiki is not instead of being able to concentrate on how effective Reiki cures can be.

[257] Dr Usui was inspired by esoteric subjects from four years of age when in a monastery.

[258] Reiki 1 spiritual rei healing.

[259] Reiki 2 material (low frequency physical) methods of curing.

[260] Reiki 2 Hatsurei ho.

[261] Reiki 1 technique of scanning with the eyes.

[262] Technique to break up a concentrated negative energy

[263] Non-touch massage allows energy from the hands to disperse wider areas of negative energy.

and other sites of swelling[264]. Chronic illnesses, however, may not be dealt with in this way[265], but I remember some cases of chronic illnesses which, usually requiring several sessions of treatment, have been successfully treated with just one session of Usui Reiki Therapy[266].

How to explain this kind of phenomenon to modern medicinal circles? The facts of the account would sound more fantastic than the contents of a novel. However, if those actively interested in the teachings take a real look at the text, I believe they will assent to the assertions of those teachings. No matter how much the wordsmith may use sophistry in his art, he cannot deride the truth[267].

Q: Cannot illness be cured without believing in the Usui Reiki Therapy?

A: Unlike psychological treatment, hypnotherapy and other mental treatments, the Usui Reiki Therapy does not bring with it empty implications[268]. It does not therefore require an explicit consent on the part of the patient[269] or any loyalty to the practitioner concerned. Not only that, we practitioners of the Usui Reiki Therapy do not mind however much our practices are doubted, held in contempt or rejected[270]. For example, the Usui Reiki Therapy is remarkably effective in treating even those who are unconscious of the world around them, such as infants and patients with

---

264 All injuries or localized illnesses may be treated by localized healing.

265 In this paragraph Dr Usui shows in-depth knowledge of healing, understanding that local injuries and all-over diseases need to be treated differently. He did not passively allow energy to flow through as taught by Mrs. Takata, nor believe that Reiki is so intelligent it knows what to do. He had many techniques, therapies and strategies, all under the heading of Usui Reiki Therapy.

266 This is true for most experienced healers. For example, I have found that arthritis, asthma, and rheumatism that normally take a number of sessions to help, have occasionally been cured in one session.

267 Dr Usui comes across as a highly educated and humble man.

268 Highly knowledgeable, Dr Usui was not averse to being blunt and tough to impart his message.

269 Contrary to many books Dr Usui says categorically that patients do not have to give permission

270 Patients do not have to believe in Reiki.

serious diseases[271]. People who believe in, admire and respect our therapy with only the first treatment, would number one in ten, if that[272]. Many such people appreciate for the first time, upon being treated once, the efficacy of the Usui Reiki Therapy, and all at once, they begin to trust it[273].

Q: What sorts of diseases are cured by the Usui Reiki Therapy?

A: A great deal of diseases, displaying mental or physical symptoms, are cured[274].

Q: Does the Usui Reiki Therapy concern itself solely with the curing of diseases?

A: No, not at all. The therapy does not involve the treatment of the body's diseases alone. It can remedy a troubled heart or anguish, imbecility or a poor constitution generally, cowardice or timidity, indecision or infirmity of purpose, nervousness, and other unfortunate conditions[275]. Further, by adopting the spirit of the teachings of Shinto and Buddhism[276], and with an eye to treating future generations[277], the results of the Usui Reiki Therapy can be that both oneself and others may be filled with happiness.

Q: What are the reasons for successful cures by means of the Usui Reiki Therapy?

---

[271] Patients do not even have to know that Reiki is being given - for Reiki still works effectively.

[272] Showing possibly a similar reaction to present-day patients.

[273] Showing how effective Reiki is after just one session.

[274] Once again the word 'cure'. Cures seem a major reason why Dr Usui promoted Reiki.

[275] Again showing that Dr Usui's main aim was to remedy all ills

[276] As Dr Usui lived in Japan, he promoted Japanese faiths to enhance Reiki healing. But, on his deathbed at the age of 27 Japanese Gods told him it is acceptable to follow other paths. So if he had taught in other countries, he may have included the faith of that country as part of Reiki.

[277] For Dr Usui, it was not enough to treat those around him – he wanted to ensure Reiki would help people long after he had gone.

A: This method of therapy was not handed down to me by several people throughout the land of Japan[278], nor did I study it in order to discover the spiritual capabilities of therapy[279]. During my period of fasting[280], I exposed myself to the atmosphere[281]. In so doing, I was wondrously inspired, and realized purely by chance[282] that I had discovered the spiritual capabilities of therapy. Therefore, as the founder of the Usui Reiki Therapy, I find it difficult to give a clear account of the therapy myself. Scholars and intellectuals are devoting themselves to the study of the therapy, and although it is difficult to draw conclusions on the basis of modern science, there will naturally come a time when the Usui Reiki Therapy will be consistent with science[283].

Q: Does Usui Reiki Therapy make use of medications, and are there not bad effects?

A: The therapy never avails itself of medical equipment. A cure is achieved solely by a steady gaze[284], or breathing[285], stroking[286], the laying

---

[278] Dr Usui states clearly that no one taught him Reiki.

[279] Here, he categorically states that he did not study to discover that Reiki works.

[280] A reference to the fasting often undertaken on Mount Kurama as a spiritual exercise?

[281] Perhaps this is a polite Japanese expression for bathing naked in Mt Kurama's open-air hot spring baths, and contemplating enlightenment. (The next sentence explains that Dr Usui received enlightenment.)

[282] Although it is known from his diaries that he was interested in metaphysical subjects for many years, Dr Usui did not deliberately search for Reiki.

[283] Dr Usui hoped that science would prove Reiki. Many properly scientific constructed studies, including my own studies, are fulfilling this prophecy.

[284] Sending Reiki through the healer's eyes into the patient's area of need.

[285] The healer blows Reiki on an area of the patient's body where energy is blocked in order to disperse the blockage.

[286] Similar to breathing, but stroking the hand in the aura just above the affected area.

on of hands[287], or light patting[288] [289].

Q: Does the Usui Reiki Therapy require medical knowledge?

A: Since our therapy is a spiritualistic method of therapy that has transcended modern science[290], it is not based on medicine. Simply, if the patient suffers pain in the chest, the practitioner of this therapy considers the patient's chest, if the stomach gives pain, then the stomach, and if there is something wrong with the eyes, then the practitioner must be concerned with the patient's eyes themselves[291]. In this way, the therapy achieves its objective of curing solely through a steady gaze on the diseased area, breathing on it, the laying-on of hands or stroking. Therefore, there is no need for the patient to take bitter medicine or be subjected to blisteringly hot moxa cautery[292], and in a short time the said diseases will be cured. This is the reason for this unique spiritualistic therapy.

Q: How do modern distinguished medical practitioners regard this therapy?

A: As far as we can see, the most distinguished of medical practitioners are giving reasonable regard to the therapy[293]. However,

---

[287] The healer places his or her hands on the patient and allows or creates correct Reiki energy.

[288] Similar to breathing and stroking, light patting just outside (not touching) a stubborn energy blocked area of the body can break up dense negative energy.

[289] This sentence shows that Dr Usui's techniques are not restricted to Mrs. Takata's system of only the laying on of hands and trusting that Reiki energy has its own intelligence.

[290] Dr Usui uses tough language. As shown below, this is based on his belief that Reiki can cure.

[291] This shows Dr Usui's deep understanding of archetypal healing. It is classic that when there is a localized pain, or a localized problem such as the eyes, the healer should never waste time giving an all-over body treatment, but should heal the localized area directly.

[292] Dr Usui believed deeply that Usui Reiki Therapy is better than 1920s Japanese medicine's.

[293] Top doctors in Japan in the 1920s were accepting Reiki

renowned medical practitioners in Europe have expressed their serious misgivings about the therapy because it does not use medications[294].

Dr Sen Nagai of the Imperial Medical University says, "As a doctor, I diagnose an illness and enter my diagnosis into the records. Although I understand the nature of the illness, I do not know how to cure it[295]."

Dr Kondo says, "One great fault of modern medicine is that, although it has made great strides, it may be described as superstition[296], and that it gives no place at all to mental function[297]."

Dr Ei Hara says, "In modern hygiene therapy, the intellect-bearing humanity of the patient is ignored, and that form of therapy has reached the stage at which the human patient is treated in the same fashion as an ordinary animal[298]. This therapy attracts great derision. I believe that in the near future, there will be a great revolution in therapy circles[299]."

Dr Rokuro Kuga says, "It is a fact that, therapies such as psychological therapy at present being practiced by non-doctors boast of brilliant achievements, whereas they are inferior to the therapy conducted by doctors[300], which relies on the type of illness concerned, the individuality of

---

294 Showing the difference between eastern and western medicine in the 1920s, with European doctors preferring to use medication as they still do today.

295 An admission that doctors can often diagnose, but rarely cure most illnesses.

296 A forceful statement that reverses the common attack against Reiki, and implies that some established medical practices are based on tradition, not evidence.

297 As today, doctors dealt only with physical problems (or separately with mental issues, and did not integrate the two processes into a system of healing the whole person.

298 Another forceful statement showing that, doctors who only treat the patient's physical symptoms are not giving credence to the mental needs or wholeness of a human being.

299 A prophesy for the current worldwide upswing in the acceptance of complementary and alternative medicine (CAM).

300 This is an atypical doctor's comment on Reiki, stated in the absence of quotable scientific research.

the patient, and the application of operations[301]. However, to blindly resist the work of the psychological therapy of non-doctors, and to strive solely to ostracize this therapy shows narrow-mindedness on the part of legitimate doctors."[302]

(Quoted from Japan Medical Bulletin)[303]

From these extracts it is indeed clear that doctors and pharmacists are beginning to recognise the efficacy[304] of these alternative forms of therapy.

Q: How does the Government view the Usui Reiki Therapy?

A: At the Budget Sectional Committee Meeting held in the House of Representatives of the Imperial Diet on 6th February 1922, Teiji Matsushita, a Member of the House of Representatives who was also a doctor of medicine[305], said, "I would like to know the Government's views on the fact that, recently, non-doctors have been curing many patients with psychological and spiritual therapies." Mr Ushio, a Government delegate, replied, "Therapies such as hypnotherapy had, until ten or twenty years before, been ridiculed. These days, however, after much scholarly research, hypnotherapy may be applied to any mental patient[306]. It is impossible to solve all aspects of the human intellect with medicine[307]. Further, doctors' work relies on what is shown by the various branches of medicine. For example, doctors suggest methods of treatment of a certain illness on the basis of medical findings. It is not, however, doctors' practice to suggest regarding all kinds of diseases that if the root of the illness is electricity,

---

[301] This is still the current medical model.

[302] Even today doctors need to have a more open mind. After all, a true scientist has an open mind to all possibilities.

[303] All the above 'distinguished medical practitioners' quotes were in the respected Japan Medical Bulletin, showing that this therapy was becoming highly regarded.

[304] To doctors and pharmacists, Reiki had an acceptable efficacy rate.

[305] To have questions asked in one of the highest institutions of the land shows governmental acceptance of the grassroots popularity of other therapies.

[306] Perhaps after ten or twenty years of research, Reiki will also be an accepted medical model.

[307] This is a governmental admission that medicine cannot help everything. Perhaps today's governments should make similar admissions?

electricity should be applied, and that if it is appropriate to touch the patient, then the doctor should go ahead and do that[308]."

Therefore, the Usui Reiki Therapy does not come under the law relating to doctors, or under the regulations to supervise acupuncture and moxa cautery[309].

Q: The Usui Reiki Therapy has the reputation that the use of its spiritual power is a natural gift, and as such, is endowed solely to specific persons. Thus, it is not something that just anybody can study and put into practice. What do you think?

A: No, not at all[310]. Any being who has received the gift of belonging to the Universe is equipped with this therapy's spiritual power as a blessing from Heaven. This is true of all phenomena: grass, trees, and the birds and the beasts. But since Man is the Lord of Creation, this spiritual power is particularly strongly manifest in human beings. This, expressed in concrete terms, has emerged in the form of the Usui Reiki Therapy[311].

Q: If that is so, can anyone be initiated into the methods of the Usui Reiki Therapy?

A: Of course[312]. From eminent scholars, both male and female[313], to the illiterate, can, if they are equipped with common sense[314], impressively cure their own diseases within a short time, and unerringly acquire the spiritual power to cure the diseases of others. Up to today, one thousand and several hundred persons have been initiated into the Usui Reiki Therapy, and not even one of these practitioners' Reiki careers has come to

---

[308] A governmental admission that doctors are limited in ability and technique.

[309] A statement by implication by Dr Usui that Reiki should have its own laws.

[310] Dr Usui is emphatic - it is not true that one needs a special gift to practice Reiki.

[311] This paragraph of beautiful language describes wonderfully the inherent capability of all people to practice Reiki.

[312] Once again, Dr Usui is emphatic in his response.

[313] Contradicting Mrs. Takata's claim that she was the only female initiated into Reiki.

[314] Intellectual or literacy capability is not needed – common sense is.

nothing[315]. Even those at the beginning of their initiation have been able impressively to exercise the spiritual powers of healing. If you care to think of it, it will seem incomprehensible that within a little time one can be endowed with the spiritual power to cure a disease, which is considered the most difficult task a person can undertake. I think that is an extremely natural reaction. However, the ability to accomplish this most difficult task with ease is the special feature of our spiritual therapy[316].

Q: If it is possible to cure other people's diseases, is it possible to cure one's own disease?

A: Why should a person who cannot cure his own disease be able to cure his own disease[317]?

Q: How would one be initiated into the more exoteric dimensions of the therapy?

A: The initiation into the more exoteric[318] side of Usui Reiki Therapy consists of the Therapy of Discovering the Spirit[319], the Tapping Therapy, the Stroking Therapy, the Therapy of Pressing with the Hands[320], the

---

[315] A statement that, given the practitioner has common sense to follow Reiki correctly, I have found to be true.

[316] Beautiful language to describe how easy it is to cure with Reiki.

[317] The translator said that he spent much time deciphering this sentence, and that this must be a Japanese conundrum.

[318] 'That is exoteric which is communicable to the outer circle of disciples.' (Fowler's Modern English Usage, Sir Ernest Gowers, Guild Publishing, 1986.)

[319] Understanding one's spiritual nature.

[320] Not allowed by most western Codes of Practice and insurance policies unless the Reiki practitioner is adequately qualified in massage or similar because of the dangers of fracturing weak bones.

Remote Therapy[321], the Natural Disposition Therapy[322], and so on[323]. The aspiring practitioner is first initiated into the elementary teachings, and then those who have achieved outstanding results, deported themselves well, and are enthusiastic, are initiated into the esoteric teachings[324].

Q: In the Usui Reiki Therapy, are there stages above the exoteric teachings?

A: There are the mystic teachings[325].

[Ends]

The text dates from 1920s and is beautifully written by a trained calligrapher. Medical quotations are in classical Japanese, which makes it a highly respectable document.[326]

---

321 Distant healing.

322 Disposition means, 'temperament; personality; a tendency.' Chambers Compact Dictionary, Chambers Harrap Publishers Ltd, 2000. Or 'setting in order, a person's natural qualities of mind and character.' The Oxford Everyday Dictionary, J.M. Hawkins and E.S.C. Weiner, The Leisure Circle Ltd, 1985. Dr Usui is stating that Reiki included a specific therapy aimed at improving these human qualities.

323 Suggesting that Dr Usui introduced many Therapies under the umbrella heading of Reiki.

324 Although Mrs. Takata's students introduced 'time gaps' between the Reiki levels, Dr Usui had 'quality gaps'. So, providing students proved their ability and understanding of what had already been taught and behaved well with common sense, and showed enthusiasm they could automatically move on to the next level. This obviously meant that good students could move on quickly, whereas not-so-good students were not allowed to move on until they portrayed these three qualities.

325 The translator said that he deliberated for much time before choosing the word 'mystic.' For higher-level Reiki practitioners, mystic has 'spiritual or occult or theological implications'. (Fowler's Modern English Usage, Sir Ernest Gowers, Guild Publishing, 1986.) Therefore, by suggestion, if exoteric meant the teachings for the outer circle of disciples, the mystic teachings were for the inner circle only. Therefore Dr Usui cannot describe the mystic teachings openly, and the document ends here.

326 Comment from the translator, the translator for the Japanese Ambassador in London.

Appendix 3

List of Morihei Tanaka's publications

1. 1910 "TAIREIDO SHINTEN"
2. 1911 "TENSHIN SIJO TAIREI SHINTEN"
3. 1916 "TAIREIDO OYOBI REISIJUTSU KOJUROKU Vol. 1-2"
4. 1918 "TAIREIDO NO HONGI"
5. 1918 "TAIREIDO SHUGENDEN"
6. 1919 "TAIREIDO, A New Revelation Showing The True System Of Life; an outline only"
7. 1920 "TAIREIDO, A New Revelation for the Spiritual, Mental and Physical Salvation of Mankind" - the book presented herein
8. 1921-22 "TAIREIDO GAKUBUMON Vol.1 - 2"
9. "TAIREIDO REISHIJUTSU KOUJUROKU Vol.1 - 2" Apparently reprinted edition of (7), published by Sengabo
10. "TAIREIDO REISHIJUTSU KOUJUROKU Vol.1 - 2" Published by Hachiman Shoten
11. And commentaries on Taireido: "TAIREIDO - Methods of developing super power" by Ikko Takagi

It is also known that Morihei Tanaka had at least one article published in at least one media, The Japan Magazine.

Appendix 4

Allan Sweeney – brief bio

Although you might not believe it if you met me now, I used to be registered as being 80% disabled. One day, I unexpectedly found I had a healing gift, curing my daughter of a damaged back and her friend of a torn ligament. Despite subsequent instantaneous cures for others, I still had illness and hospitalizations. Afraid of being laughed at or thought of as having ego, I did not advertise, and healing ability was hidden even from my family.

Then my adrenals collapsed, severe osteoporosis developed, and a prognosis was given of 2 years to live. Whilst dying, a sudden realization came that I should have offered healing and teaching much more. A deep promise was made to my soul that, given another chance, I would do it properly. Days later, in a mystical meeting, a healer cured me of life-long disablement.

Since then, beautiful things happened, including international teaching, a Harley Street Clinic, doing research for ADD, ADHD, cancer, fractures, anger, sadness, depression, pain, deafness, eyesight, tinnitus, back pain etc; being on various committees including the Doctor-Healer Network, the British Psychological Society, and the UK House of Commons Parliamentary Group for Complementary and Alternative Medicine; and my 10-bed residential Reiki, Therapy and Teaching Centre on the beach in Margate UK, which is blessed to have had so many amazing students and patients.
For further information please see

http://usuisteacher.com

Or my site http://reiki-healing.com

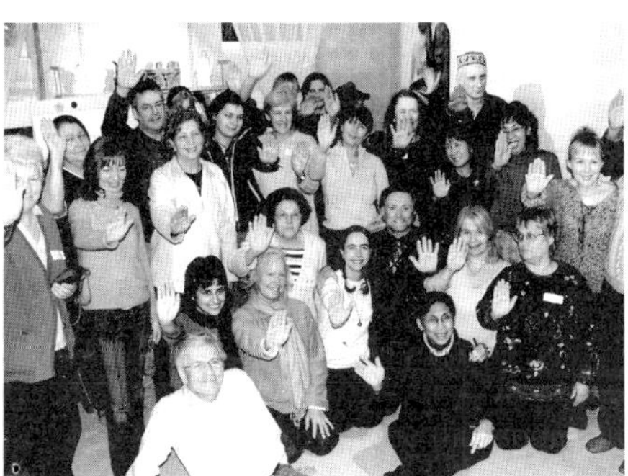

A Reiki Master Teacher's Class at the residential centre 'Heaven-by-the-Sea', Margate (Allan Sweeney is kneeling, 3rd from right)

Appendix 5

Frank Shortt - brief bio

I was born in 1978, in Stavanger Norway, and always had a taste for spiritual and cultural studies. I was especially fond of Eastern thought and philosophy and studied them widely.

In UK during the period while at University (1997-2003), I practiced Tai Chi and Shaolin Kung Fu (then: Ving Tsun, from 2004-date). I avidly studied all the esoteric and mystical teachings I found at the University Library, and started looking for a practical approach to all these teachings; this is when I met Allan Sweeney who guided me through the teachings of Usui-sensei, and the practice of Reiki Ryoho/Reiho.

His courses were deeply insightful both spiritually and in terms of practical treatment for different conditions, and have been a great asset of knowledge to pass within the family and friends, who all have benefited from it. Experiencing that this practice has the ability to relieve chronic conditions like rheumatic joints, arthritis, cancer, nerve-damage, headache, cuts etc etc has helped me and my extended family greatly the last 10 years. I only wish I had come by this system at an earlier age.

As a Reiki practitioner and an avid student of oriental spiritual subjects, I have for many years researched and discussed topics pertaining to Reiki history, as well as its symbology and practices relating to Japanese historical & modern spiritual practices and disciplines.

My professional work has allowed me to explore many cultures around the globe, and I am both honored and privileged to have spent several weeks in Japan, both in 2006 and again in 2008, during which time we spent much time learning about the intricacies of Shinto/Buddhist history from a professor in Kyoto, and Tokyo. Both Kyoto and Tokyo have beautiful shrines and temples where we spent days filming.

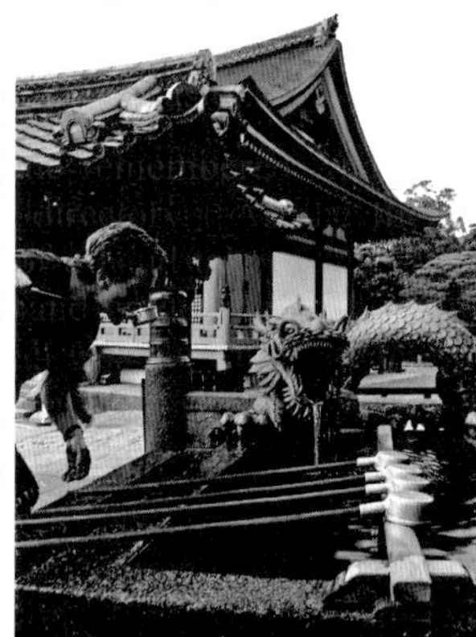

Frank Shortt
honoring the pure water at
Kiyomizu-dera Temple, Kyoto

For more information please visit the website for this book:
http://usuisteacher.com
Or my site: http://reiki-ho.org